1 Frontiers in European Radiology

Editors-in-Chief

A.L. Baert · E. Boijsen
W.A. Fuchs · F.H.W. Heuck

Springer-Verlag
Berlin Heidelberg New York 1982

Professor Dr. Albert L. Baert

Universitaire Ziekenhuizen, Department of Diagnostic Radiology,
Capucijnenvoer 35, B-3000 Leuven

Professor Dr. Erik Boijsen

University Hospital, Department of Diagnostic Radiology, S-22185 Lund

Professor Dr. Walter A. Fuchs

Inselspital Bern, Institut für Diagnostische Radiologie der Universität,
CH-3010 Bern

Professor Dr. Friedrich H. W. Heuck

Radiologisches Institut im Zentrum Radiologie, Katharinenhospital
(Lehrkrankenhaus der Universität Tübingen),
Kriegsbergstr. 60, D-7000 Stuttgart

With 113 Figures (in 187 Separate Illustrations)

ISBN-13: 978-3-642-95392-7 e-ISBN-13: 978-3-642-95390-3
DOI: 10.1007/978-3-642-95390-3

Softcover reprint of the hardcover 1st edition 1982

2121/3130-543210

Preface

The dramatic evolution of new technology in diagnostic and therapeutic radiology has changed the whole field of medicine. Ultrasonography, computed tomography, nuclear magnetic resonance, and digital radiography are those new techniques which are undergoing continuous development, providing us with increasingly refined methods for establishing the cause of disease and for treating the patient. Using radiologic technique, ingenious methods are continuously being developed to ensure less expensive, less traumatic, and more efficient therapy. Transluminal angioplasty, embolization of tumors or bleeding vessels, extraction or dissolution of stones, and regional infusions are some of these therapeutic methods in modern diagnostic radiology.

Every day new ideas arise which are published in a multitude of papers. This heavy flow of information limits the possibility of selecting from a core of information and often prevents radiologists from communicating efficiently with their colleagues in other countries or continents. European radiologists are additionally hampered from participating in international communication because of the language barriers created by the national journals. As a result, Europe's contribution to scientific progress in this interdisciplinary field has influenced only regional developments.

The series Frontiers in European Radiology will provide a forum for (mainly) European scientists in clinical and experimental radiology. Young radiologists in many European countries work on a specific project and present their research in a variety of journals. For their major works they frequently make a comprehensive review in their national language both of their own work and of the work of others in the same field. We hold the opinion that these reviews, as well as additional unpublished work, should be available to all who want to keep abreast in the field of radiology. For this purpose we have chosen a book series rather than a journal since this enables such reports to be presented in far greater depth. We thus intend that Frontiers in European Radiology should become a concise source of detailed information for those wanting to keep up-to-date with scientific progress in the field. The papers presented in this volume demonstrate the wide range of topics this series aims to cover. We hope that we can thus provide readers with topical information which will be of use to him in his day-to-day work. Indeed, we hope that we can achieve even more, namely to improve communication between radiologists from all countries irrespective of language.

The Editors

Contents

Percutaneous Extraction of Renal Calculi

I. Fernström and B. Johansson [1]

1 Introduction

Rupel and *Brown* in 1941 described extraction of a residual postoperative renal calculus. Under general anaesthesia, a nephrostomy canal from the previous operation allowed stone removal using a panendoscope and a pair of grasping forceps. Three additional cases using a similar technique were reported in 1974 by *Bissada* et al. (one case) and by *Brantly* and *Shirley* (two cases). Three recent papers report success using a fluoroscopic method instead of a panendoscope (*Karamcheti* and *Donell* 1977; *Palestrant* et al. 1980; *Hellsten* et al. 1980). In one of these patients a special stone trapping device, said to have superior merits to the usual Dormia basket, had been constructed (*Hellsten* et al. 1980). As we have had considerable experience in both percutaneous nephrostomy (*Almgård* and *Fernström* 1974) and non-operative extraction of retained bile duct stones with the technique described by *Burhenne* (1973), it seemed logical to attempt extraction of renal calculi via a nephrostomy canal. Renal calculi tend to recur and sometimes

1 Departments of Diagnostic Radiology and Urology, Karolinska Hospital, S-10401 Stockholm

necessitate renal surgery which, because of postoperative fibrosis, can be difficult and not always free from complications. We therefore regard percutaneous extraction as being primarily indicated in patients with high operative risk and in those who previously had had stones surgically removed. The first extraction was performed at Karolinska Hospital in 1974. The method avoids operative mobilisation of the kidney to perform a nephrostomy, but instead uses the technique of percutaneous puncture of the renal pelvis, under stereotactic radiological control, and gradual dilatation of the canal until it is wide enough for the stone to be removed. Although successful reports of our first three cases were published in 1976 (*Fernström* and *Johansson*), *Boyce* in 1978 Yearbook of Urology said, "Nephrostomy or pyelostomy tubes in the removal of renal calculi should be regarded as disasters." We feel this commentary is inaccurate in the light of our publications since 1976 (*Andersson* and *Fernström* 1977; *Fernström* and *Johansson* 1980). It is therefore of some importance that we now collect, edit, and summarise our results.

2 Materials and Methods

Percutaneous extraction has been performed on a total of 39 patients for renal calculi and on 4 further patients for other reasons, making a total of 43 cases. These 4 patients included 3 with renal candidosis and 1 with calcification within the renal parenchyma, but as the initial reason for nephrostomy was suspected calculus, these are also included. Age distribution was as follows: 12 cases under 45, 14 between 45 and 60, and 17 over 60 years of age. There were 24 males and 19 females. Both age and sex distribution correspond to that normally seen in patients with renal calculi.

The indications for percutaneous pyelonephrostomy were: 29 cases with recurrent or residual stones after previous surgery, 7 patients not considered operable because of cardiac or pulmonary disease and 7 patients for whom, because of size and position of the calculus, a percutaneous method was considered more suitable than surgery.

Included in the material are 6 patients who had an intracalyceal calculus of less than 10 mm diameter which did not appear to obstruct flow. It seemed, therefore, strange that these patients had so much renal pain, radiating to the groin and genitalia, and one questions the relationship between these small stones and patients' symptoms. Most of the patients had a long history of renal stones and those 28 patients with more than 5 years' symptoms included 15 with troublesome stones for more than a decade. Stones greater than 20 mm in diameter were not considered suitable for percutaneous extraction. At the time of treatment 32 patients had a single calculus, while 7 had two or more; the total number of stones was 50, of which 18 were situated in a calyx, 23 in the renal pelvis and 9 in the ureter. Six of the 39 patients underwent operation for removal of their renal stones, but when one or more could not be located, a pyelonephrostomy tube was inserted towards completion of the operation. An attempt was then made to remove the residual stones at the Department of Radiology.

The technique used is similar to that for a normal percutaneous nephrostomy, but the canal must be widened sufficiently for insertion of forceps or a Dormia stone basket to remove the calculus during fluoroscopy. The patient is fully conscious throughout the whole procedure, but analgesics are given if required. All stages, including insertion of nephrostomy tube, dilatation and removal of the calculi, were performed by one physician in order to gain experience and improve his technique.

Renal drainage by percutaneous nephrostomy is now a standard method of treatment, with more than 500 successful cases at the Department of Radiology, Karolinska Hospital, Stockholm, and has been fully described previously (*Andersson* and *Fernström* 1977). Working together with AB Meda[1], we have now developed a complete cutaneous nephrostomy kit in order to improve and simplify the procedure.

The following points should be carefully studied before extraction is attempted:

2.1 Renal Pelvis Anatomy in Relation to the Stone

A high dose of contrast medium (1 cc 76% contrast medium/kg body wt.) shows pelvic anatomy and allows excellent localisation of the stone if oblique and lateral projections are included. When renal function is poor, an antegrade pyelography immediately prior to the nephrostomy is recommended.

2.2 Position of the Nephrostomy Canal

When only renal draining is required, a normal percutaneous nephrostomy may be performed at any suitable site, as long as the renal pelvis is penetrated dorsolaterally. For calculus removal, however, the canal ought to be so angled as to allow instrumentation directly towards the stone.

2.3 Technique of Pelvic Puncture

It is essential that the line of puncture runs approximately straight to that part of the pelvis or calix previously selected. This is facilitated by the use of fluoroscopy in two planes, which also acts as a pathfinder and thus minimises pelvic damage and the risk of puncture of the renal artery or vein. If the pelvis is not already dilated, the whole procedure is simplified by first using a fine calibre needle to enter the renal pelvis, which is then filled with contrast medium. The resulting dilatation of the pelvis and calyces allows exact penetration with a wider bore tube.

2.4 Dilatation of the Nephrostomy Canal

Using a similar method to that described previously (*Andersson* and *Fernström* 1977), a wide polythene tube is inserted into the canal, using a suitable guide wire, on each or alternate days. The final anticipated dilatation will depend on the

---

1 AB Meda, Box 138, S-490 22 Gothenburg

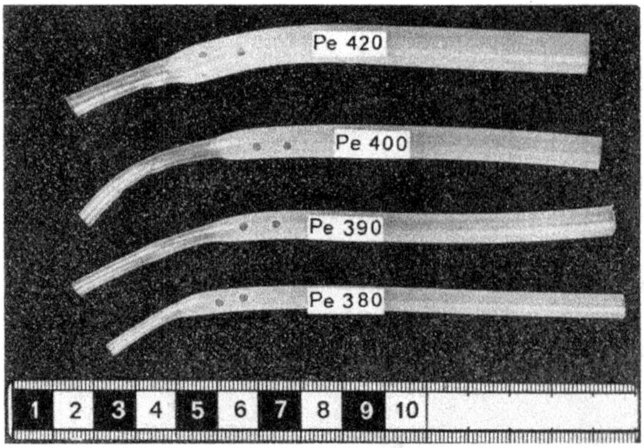

Fig. 1. Wide bore polythene tubes used for dilatation

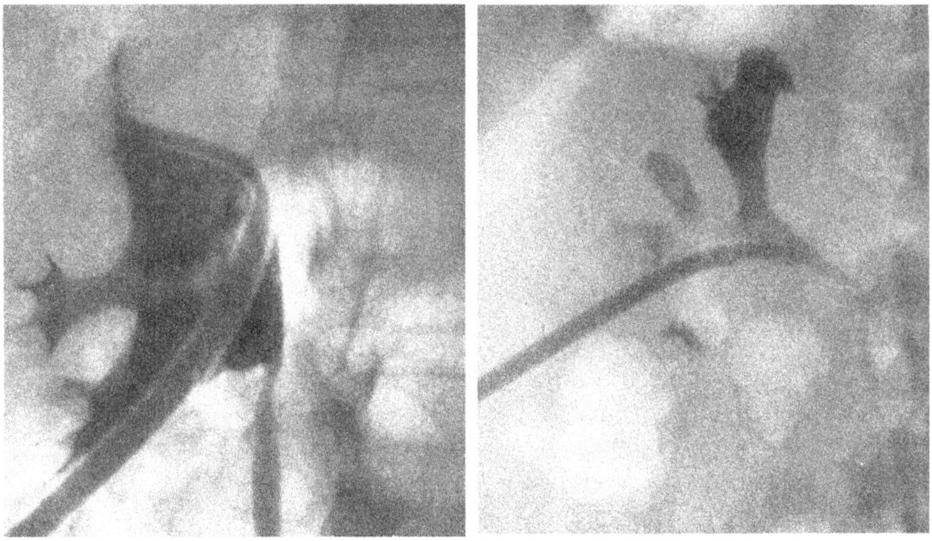

Fig. 2a, b. Various tube positions following dilatation for subcutaneous stone extraction. **a** The (Pe 420) tapered curved tip of the tube lying in an upper calyx; **b** the (Pe 390) tapered curved tip of the tube at the pelviureteric junction

estimated diameter of the calculus. Those dilator tubes not found in the nephrostomy kit correspond to the following diameters: Tube Pe 380 = 5.95 mm, Pe 390 = 6.68 mm, Pe 400 = 7.80, and Pe 420 = 9.70 mm (Fig. 1).

2.5 Dilator Tubes' Outer Diameter and Calculus Size

The total extraction diameter corresponds to that of the stone plus the width of the extracting instrument around the stone. It is not, however, essential to dilate the canal to this diameter or even to that of the stone alone. Dilatation to at least Pe 380 will avoid difficulty with insertion of the various extracting instruments.

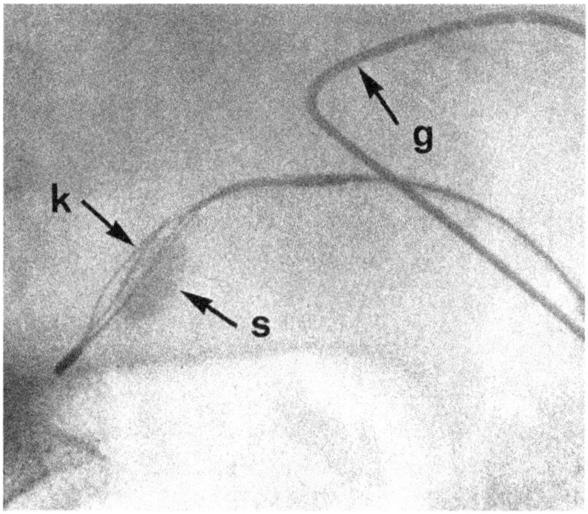

Fig. 3. Percutaneous extraction of a 15 mm renal pelvic stone. "Reserve guide wire" in position with its tip in an upper calyx. *s*, stone; *k*, Dormia stone basket; *g*, reserve guide wire

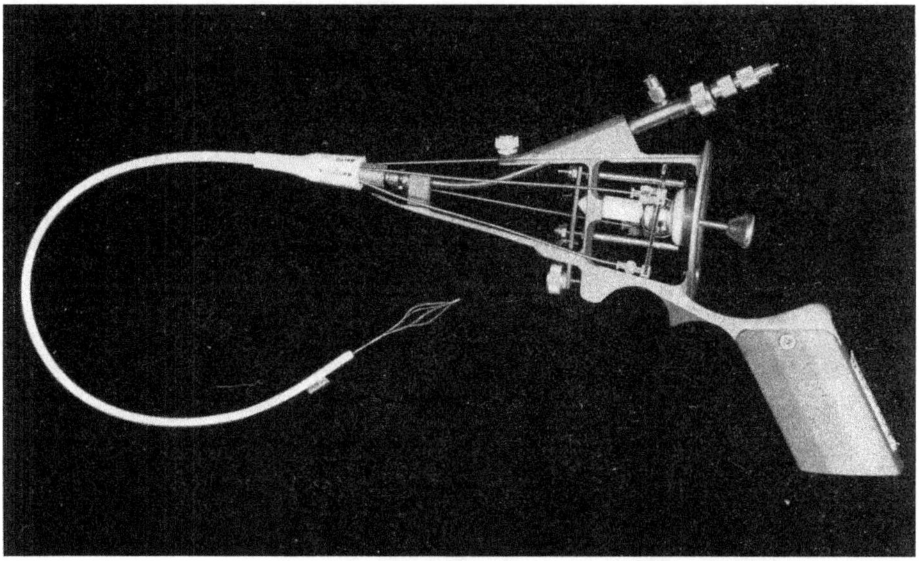

Fig. 4. Selector instrument and an inserted open Dormia basket

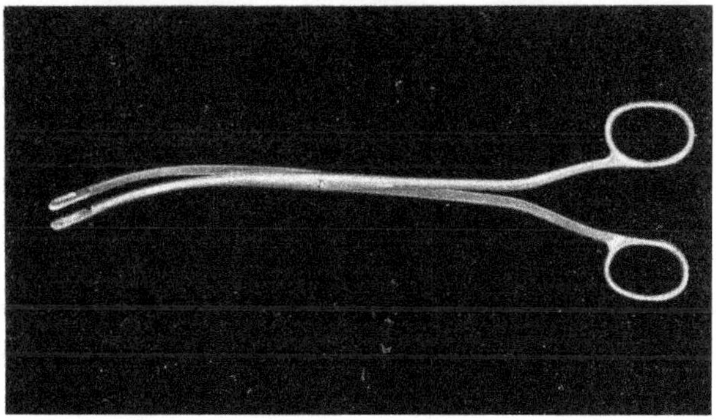

Fig. 5. Randall forceps

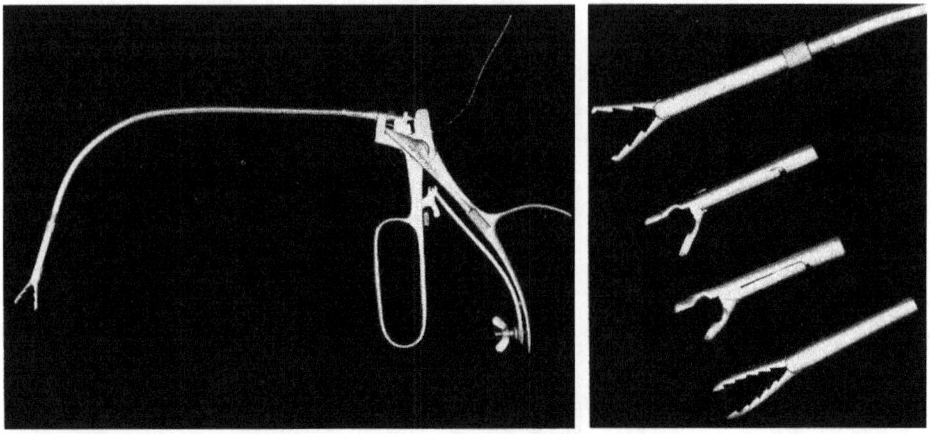

a b

Fig. 6. a Stone removal forceps with fixed stem and exchangeable jaws; **b** selection of the exchangeable jaws

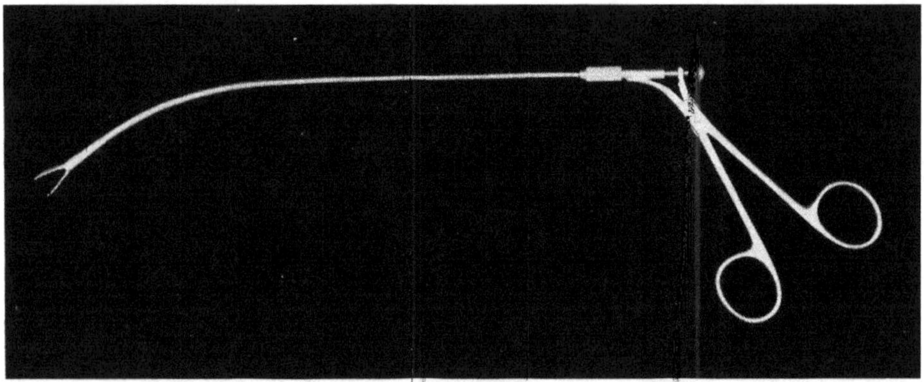

Fig. 7. Stone removal forceps with flexible stem and fixed jaws ("Pfau")

Fig. 8a–d. A postoperatively retained stone can be removed after a few days via a nephrostomy canal. **a** Post-operative film showing two larger pelvic and one small calyx (*arrow*) stone. **b** Pelvic stone extracted at first attempt, but the calyx stone (*arrow*) still present. **c** Stone (*arrow*) is reached with a curved catheter and guide wire. **d** Polythene tube (160) threaded over the guide wire is used to shift the stone into the renal pelvis with a forced saline jet. Position of catheter and anatomy visualised after injection of 5 cc contrast. *Arrows,* the two lower calyces; *u,* ureter ►

Fig. 9a, b. A 43-year-old male was a poor operative risk because of previous pulmectomy on the left, lobectomy on the right, and left-sided nephrectomy, for tuberculosis. He had severe right flank pain but urography was normal except for a 4 mm stone in the upper calyx. The pain radiated into his testicle and in order to relieve the pain a right-sided orchidectomy was performed without any effect. He was then referred to a neurosurgical unit for dorsal root division because he was unable to work and used strong analgesics. Before this treatment an attempt at percutaneous stone removal was made. The small calyx stone is pushed into the renal pelvis by a dorsally inserted needle (not shown). **a** Stone in upper medial calyx (*s*). Selector catheter directed towards upper calyx (*e*). Reserve guide wire tube at lower calyx (*arrow*). **b** Contrast medium injected to visualise the intrapelvic anatomy. Stone (*arrow*) is in an upper medial calyx ►

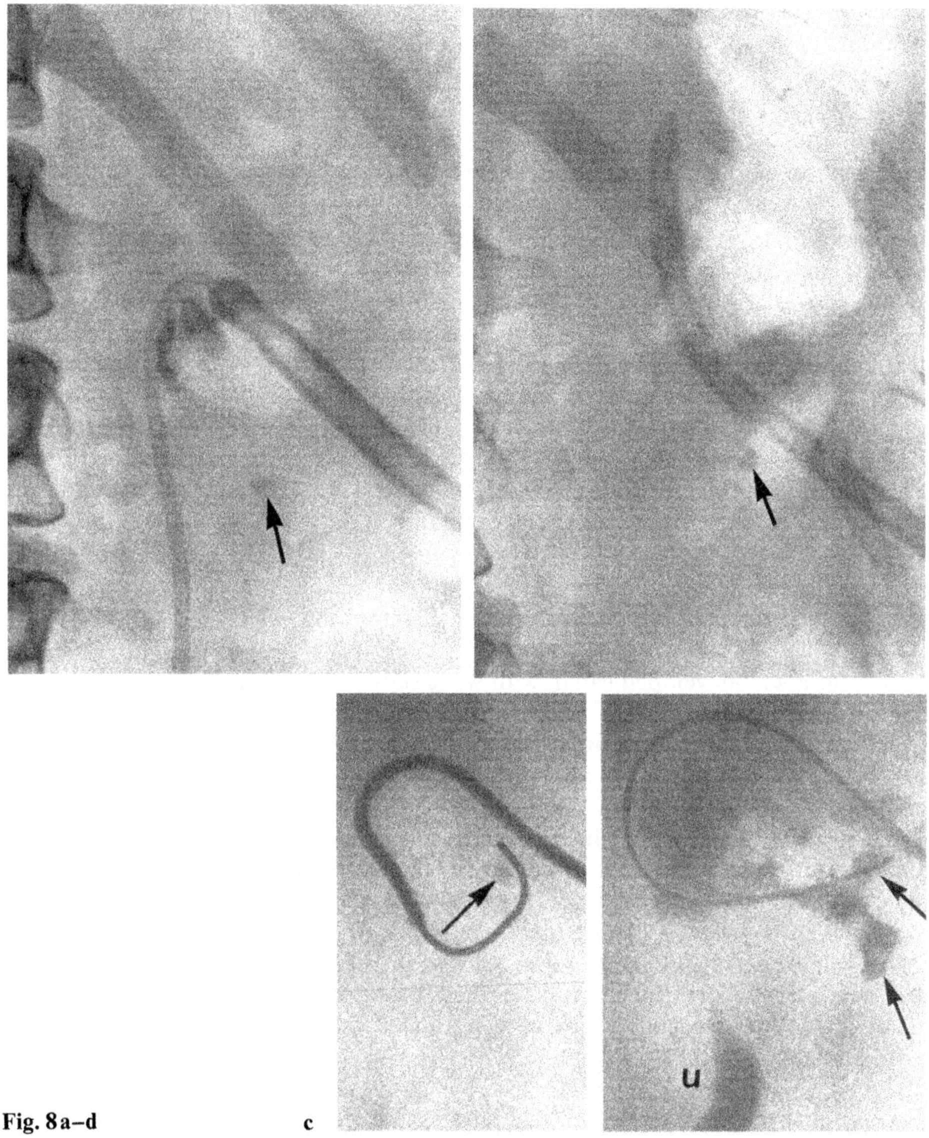

Fig. 8a–d

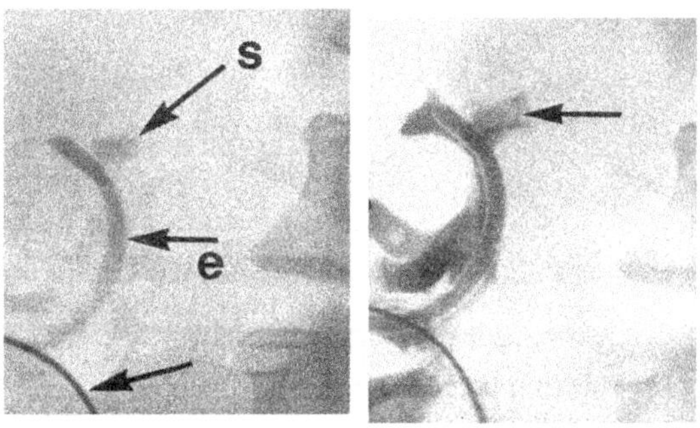

Fig. 9a, b

Stones with a diameter of 10 mm can be removed after dilatation with a Pe 390 tube but those with a diameter approaching 20 mm require canal dilatation with wider tubes.

2.6 Position of the Dilator Tube Within the Renal Pelvis

Because of their rigidity, wider calibre tubes must be inserted with greater care to avoid damage and haemorrhage to the pelvic wall.

The operator should fashion these tubes to suit the anatomy, the stone and the best position for the tip in each individual patient. The tube can be softened by steam heating to allow elongation and bending. That portion of the tube which will lie in the canal leading up to the pelvis must retain its initial outer diameter to perform adequate dilatation. The end of the tube within the pelvis should be 3–4 cm long and perforated with several side holes, and its tip may lie either in one of the calyces or at the pelvi-ureteric junction (see Fig. 2). Even if the wide calibre tubes appear to be firmly lodged in the canal they should be fixed to the skin.

2.7 When Should Stone Withdrawal Be Attempted

As soon as a well-developed canal, with walls stable enough to allow the passage of catheters or instruments, has been formed an attempt at calculus extraction is permitted. These conditions are usually fulfilled after a week, but smaller stones may be removed even earlier. Should the newly-formed canal wall be damaged by an ill-timed, injudicious or incompetent attempt at withdrawal, it may prove impossible to pass a catheter or instrument into the renal pelvis. When the dilatation time is short or there is a large discrepancy between the canal and stone diameters, canal wall damage can easily occur. Under these circumstances a "reserve guide wire" should be inserted. Before any attempt at extraction is made, a guide wire is passed via the canal so that the soft tip lies in the upper end of the ureter or at the periphery of a calyx (Fig. 3). This is retained during extraction attempts and should canal wall damage occur, it can be refashioned via the guide wire, allowing a second attempt after 2–3 days.

2.8 Catching the Calculus

All stones were caught and extracted with a Dormia stone basket or an array of forceps and scoops.

1. Both 4- and 6-wire Dormia baskets, without their elongated tapered tips, were used and inserted with the assistance of a "Selector" (Fig. 4) which assisted direction of the basket to, or even beyond, the calculus. In a few cases, however, the basket was steered into position using a pre-curved catheter.
2. Several types of forceps were used:
   a) Randall forceps (Fig. 5)

b) Stone removal forceps with fixed stem and exchangeable jaws (Fig. 6)
c) Stone removal forceps with flexible stem and fixed jaws – "Pfau" (Fig. 7)

There is generally no difficulty in catching the renal pelvic calculus using one of the above-mentioned instruments, but care must be taken to avoid damage to the pelvic wall. Laying the patient in a prone position will sometimes help in difficult cases, but calculi situated distally within a calyx may be inaccessible if the stone cannot be first eased into the pelvis. This is accomplished using a selector instrument or pre-curved catheter (Cobra, Michaelsson) to approach the calculus and by means of a saline jet or careful manipulation force the stone to fall into the pelvis (Fig. 8). As a final resort, a long, small-calibre needle can be inserted to harpoon the stone and push it into the pelvis. Fluoroscopy and a gas-filled colon help to avoid perforating the pleura and intestine (Figs. 9, 10). As the patient is fully conscious, it is possible to use pain and discomfort as an indicator of pelvic wall trauma. Severe pain precedes pelvic wall damage and incipient perforation. If renal pelvic perforation does occur, haemorrhage may result but this is unusual. Nevertheless, smaller perforations with mild haemorrhage sometimes occur but seldom necessitate abandoning the attempt at extraction. Tenderness of the renal pelvis varies from patient to patient, some feel hardly anything, while others feel each instrument movement within the pelvis. An estimation of the degree of individual renal pelvis tenderness made during the dilatation procedure can be used as a basis for avoiding perforation during operation.

Bile duct scoops are sometimes useful for shifting calculi into the pelvis. Filling the pelvis with air, provided there is no haemorrhage, will facilitate the detection of small stones (Fig. 11).

Stones within the ureter can be caught in a Dormia basket which is manoeuvred beyond the stone, opened and then, with extreme caution, slowly withdrawn (Fig. 12). Sometimes all efforts to change the position of the stone fail because of oedema of the ureteric wall. As the basket is slowly withdrawn the stone appears to move a few centimetres, however, this may not be due to its dislocation but to stretching of the ureter distal to the stone – the "concertina effect" (Fig. 13).

2.9 Calculus Extraction from the Renal Pelvis

Withdrawal seldom posses any problem when the canal is wide and the stone small (Fig. 14). If, on the other hand, these two factors are less favorable, it may be difficult for the stone and instrument to pass through the canal, and a powerful and sustained tension for as long as 15 min may be necessary before the stone is finally delivered. At this stage it is permissible to use considerably greater force than during extraction from the ureter and pelvis. The procedure is often painful and may necessitate i.v. analgesia. It is usually fairly easy to extract the stone through renal parenchyma but resistance is encountered when scars from previous surgery or muscle or fascial planes are negotiated. A narrow knife passed into the canal to cut alongside the extraction instrument has occasionally proved useful (Fig. 15). As previously emphasised, it is wise to have a reserve guide wire in position if extraction difficulties are anticipated.

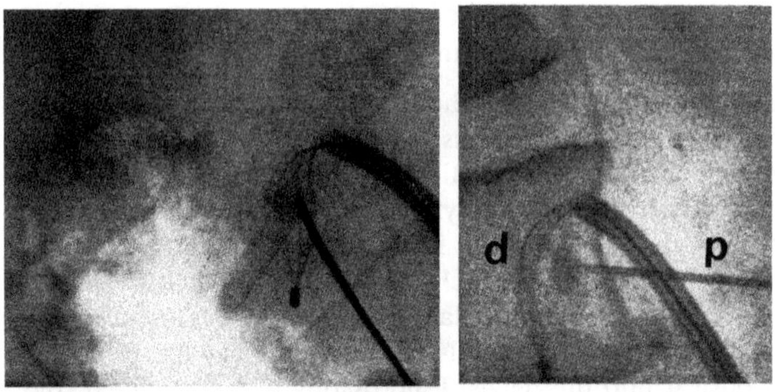

Fig. 10 a, b

a b

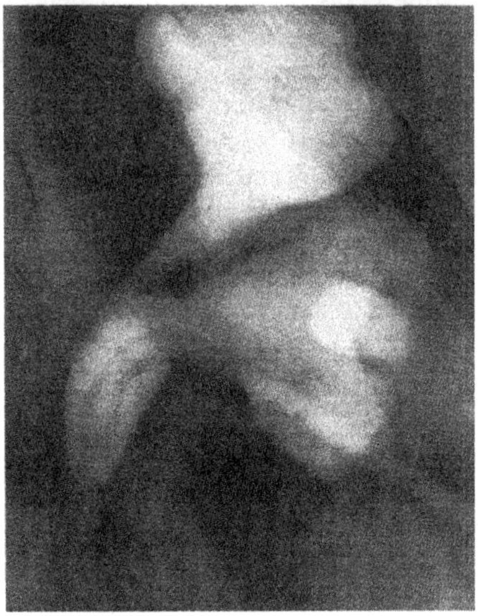

Fig. 11

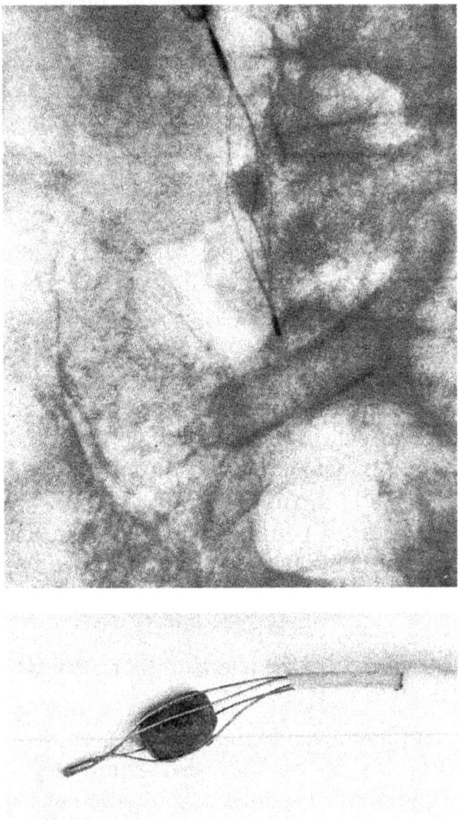

a

Fig. 12 a, b b

Fig. 10 a, b. A small calculus, harpooned via the abdomen, is pushed into the Dormia basket. **a** Frontal projection; **b** side projection (*d*, Dormia basket; *p*, harpooning needle)

Fig. 11. Following extraction of a small renal pelvic calculus, the pelvis is filled with air to confirm that no further stones are present

Fig. 12 a, b. Patient with a solitary right kidney and a dilated pelvis due to a calculus. Surgery failed to locate the stone and left the patient with a pelvic fistula. Percutaneous nephrostomy was followed after 7 days by removal of the stone, here situated in the ureter. **a** Ureteric stone caught in a Dormia basket; **b** the stone after removal

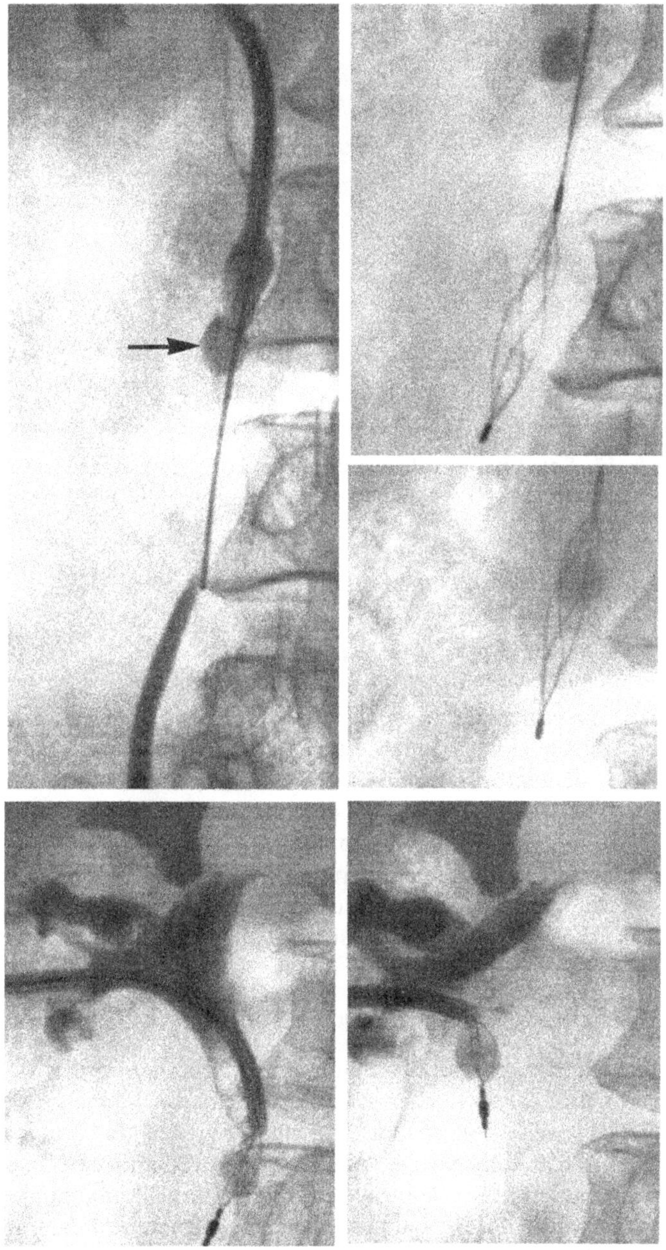

Fig. 13a–e. Ureteric stone, easily caught in a Dormia basket but resisting extraction; **a** Selector catheter reaches the stone as a closed Dormia basket passes by (*arrow,* stone); **b** Dormia basket opened beyond the stone; **c** basket encircles the stone; **d** stone is caught in the basket; **e** "concertina effect" at attempted withdrawal

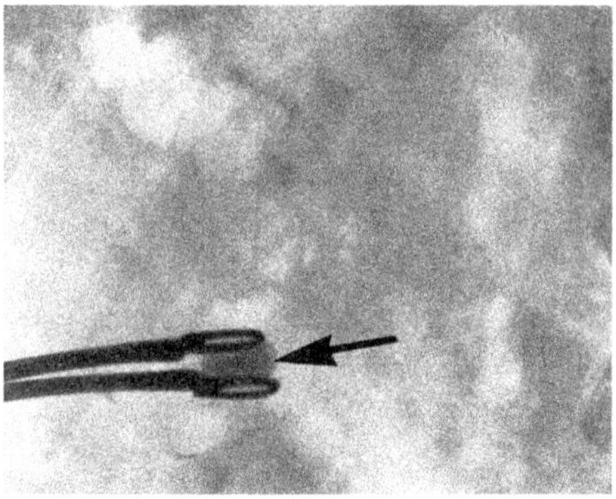

Fig. 14

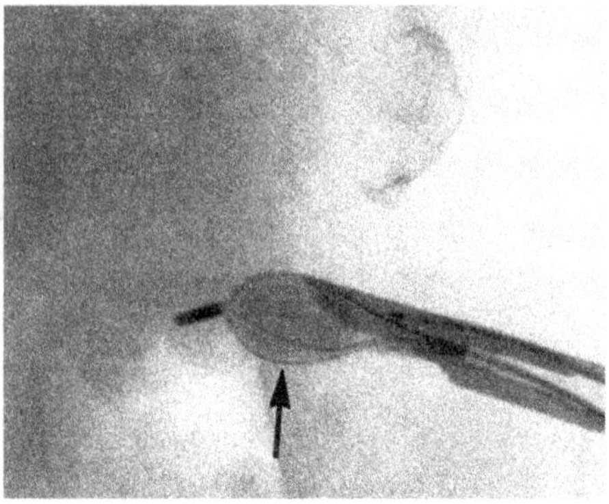

Fig. 15

Fig. 14. Renal pelvis calculus (*arrow*) caught with a pair of forceps just prior to extraction

Fig. 15. Renal pelvis calculus caught in a Dormia stone basket. Difficult delivery via the canal alleviated by longitudinal incision. The knife point can be seen close by the stone (*arrow*)

2.10 Multipe or Fragmented Stones

It is advantageous to remove all stones in the same session, but occasionally the wall of the canal is unable to tolerate the increased instrumentation. Under these circumstances insertion of a new tube of suitable diameter and a delay of two days is recommended before further extraction is attempted.

Sometimes a stone fragments within the renal pelvis or canal during extraction (Figs. 16–18) and thus may prolong or multiply the sessions. Some of the fragments can be washed out via the canal, and some through the ureter into the bladder; some, however, will require subsequent instrumental extraction (Fig. 19).

2.11 Foley Catheter Drainage Following Extraction

Following successful extraction, it is advisable to drain the renal pelvis for a day or two with a 10 or 12 Charrière Foley catheter. To confirm the patency of the ureter and absence of blood clots and small retained fragments antegrade pyelography is recommended before the catheter is removed and the patient discharged.

In a few cases computerised tomography and angiography have been used before and after extraction to ascertain the extent of haemorrhage within or outside the kidney. No bleeding could be identified (Fig. 20).

2.12 Follow-up

All the patients were examined at the Department of Urology, Karolinska Hospital and subjected to urography 6 months, 1 year and 2 years after successful stone extraction.

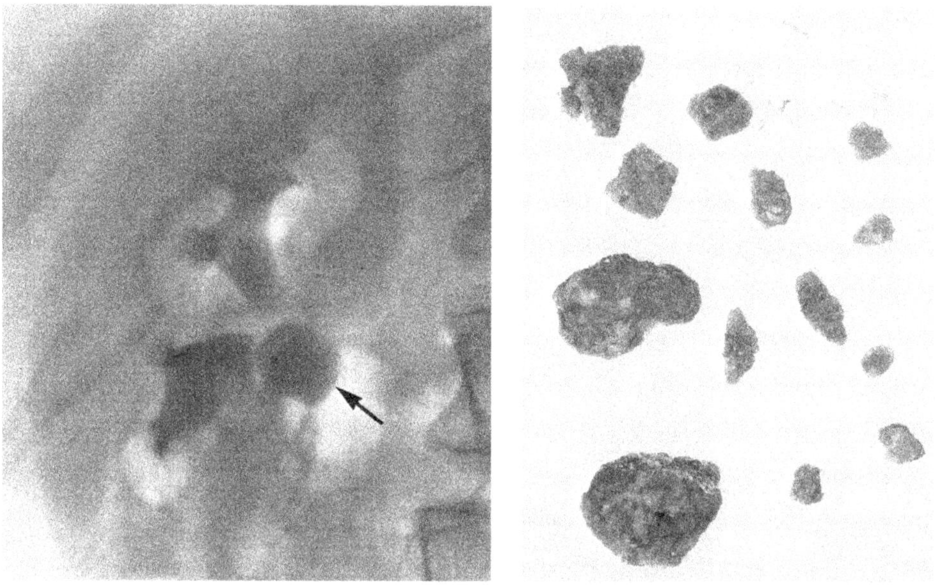

a b

Fig. 16 a, b. A renal pelvis calculus which, during an extraction attempt, has broken into 13 fragments which can all be removed at the same session. **a** Urography a week prior to treatment. A stone (*arrow*) fills the renal pelvis. **b** Removed fragments

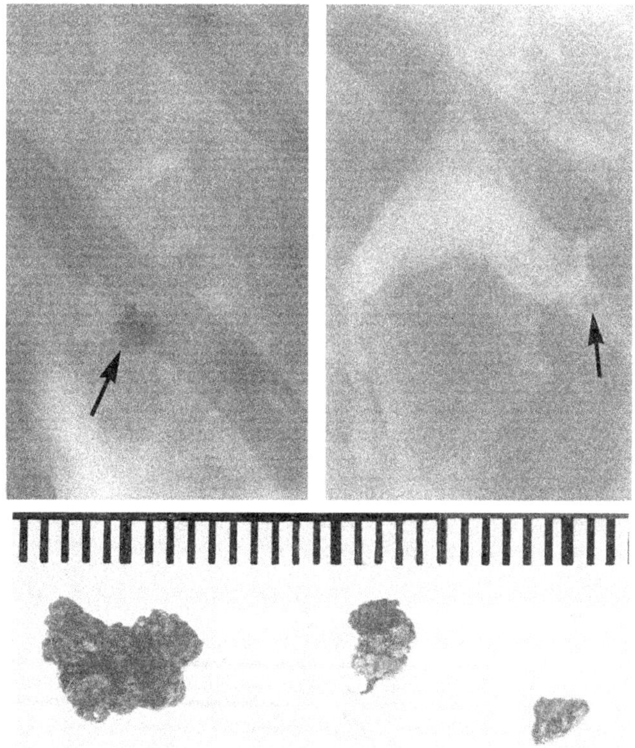

a b c

Fig. 17 a–c. During extraction a renal calculus broke into three fragments within the pelvis. The two larger fragments are removed at the first session whereas the smallest cannot be extracted until 3 days later. **a** Stone prior to extraction (*arrow*). **b** After the first extraction session a small fragment remains in a lower lateral calyx. It can be seen clearly when the pelvis is filled with air (*arrow*). **c** The three removed fragments

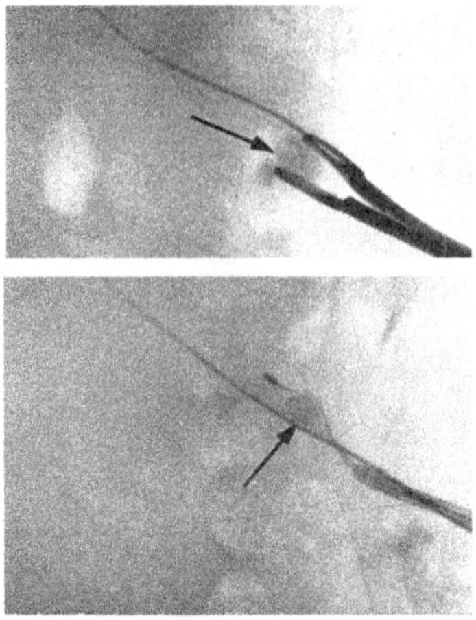

a b

Fig. 18. **a** Stone (*arrow*) being extracted from the renal pelvis with forceps (observe the reserve guide wire). It broke in two and a part remains in the canal. **b** The retained fragment (*arrow*) removed with a Dormia basket

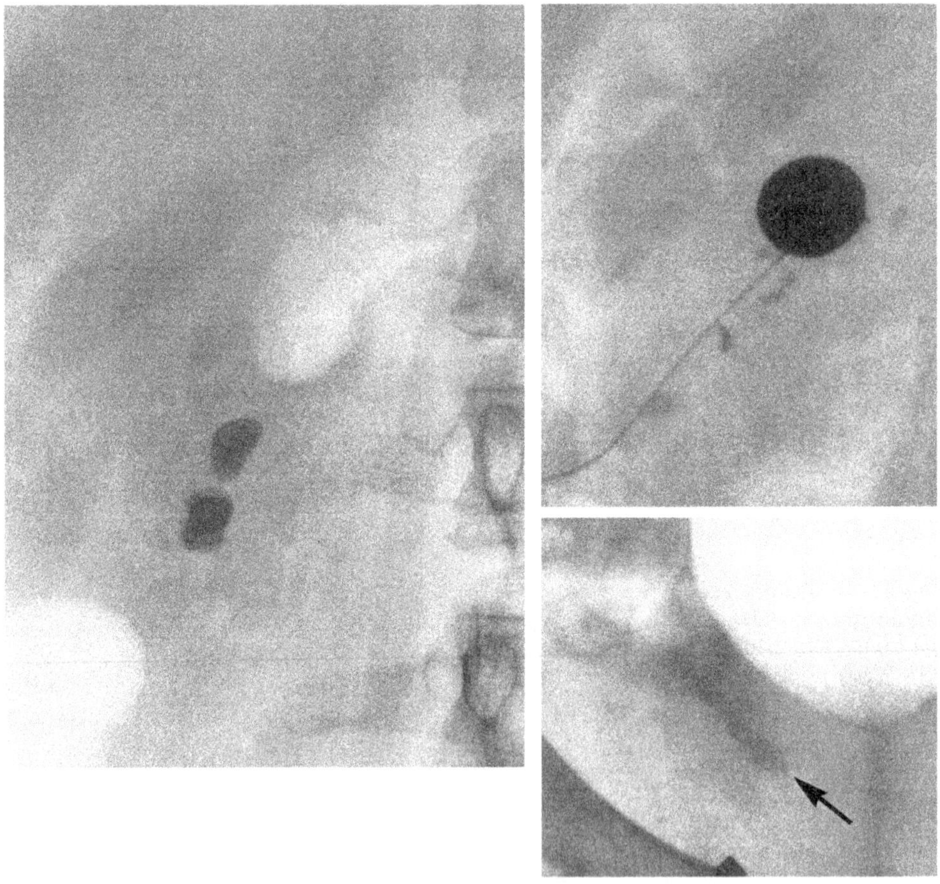

a b c

Fig. 19. **a** Case of twin stones, each 1 cm in diameter, one in a calyx, the other in the renal pelvis, requiring three extractions for complete success. The pelvic stone was easily removed with a Dormia basket but that in the calyx broke up and it took some time before all the fragments could be removed. **b** Fragments in a calyx, pelvis, and sinus tract (Foley catheter in position). **c** Fragments in the distal end of the ureter (*arrow*)

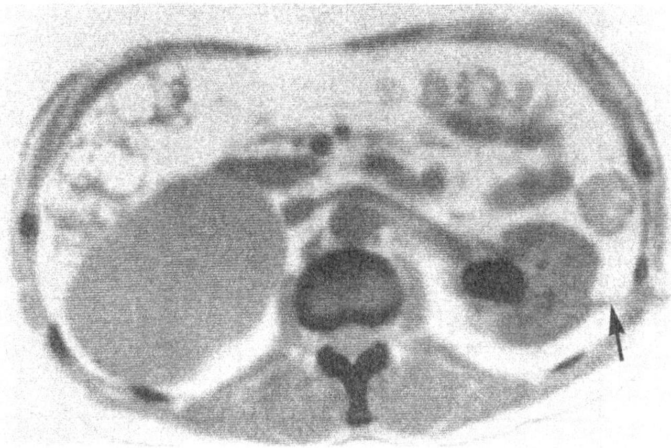

Fig. 20. Computerised tomography 1 day after difficult extraction of a large renal pelvic calculus. Foley catheter is seen (*arrow*), but there is no sign of haemorrhage in or around the kidney

3 Results

Although widely variable, the average time required for canal dilatation to a suitable size was 7 days (see Fig. 21).

Figure 22 shows the duration from percutaneous nephrostomy to complete stone removal or acknowledgement of failure. The first extraction attempt was usually performed within a day or so of final dilatation. If further sessions were required, they were interspaced with 1–2 days of rest. The patients were kept in hospital for the extraction procedures and the total length of hospitalisation varied from 11 to 41 days, with an average of 17 days. This is somewhat in excess of that shown in Fig. 22, the difference depending on those few days the stone-free kidney was drained with a Foley catheter and antegrade pyelography performed. With normal pyelography the catheter was removed and the patient discharged.

The maximum diameter of the dilated canal prior to extraction is shown in Fig. 23. Most stones can be removed through a canal following dilatation with a 390 tube (diameter about 7 mm).

The results of extraction of some 50 stones are shown in Table 1. Here the positions of the stones are given, differentiating between primary nephrostomy extraction and extraction of postoperative residual stones.

While 39 calculi could be withdrawn, 11 had to be completely or partially left behind. The primary cases, in which percutaneous nephrostomy was planned to remove a stone lying in a calyx or renal pelvis, were successful in 30 of 32 calculi, i.e. 96%. When, however, the stone was in the ureter or had to be removed via an operatively inserted nephrostomy, the success rate was reduced to about 50%.

Stones with an estimated diameter of less than 20 mm did not affect the outcome, as shown in Figs. 24 and 25. Although some suggest that stones should

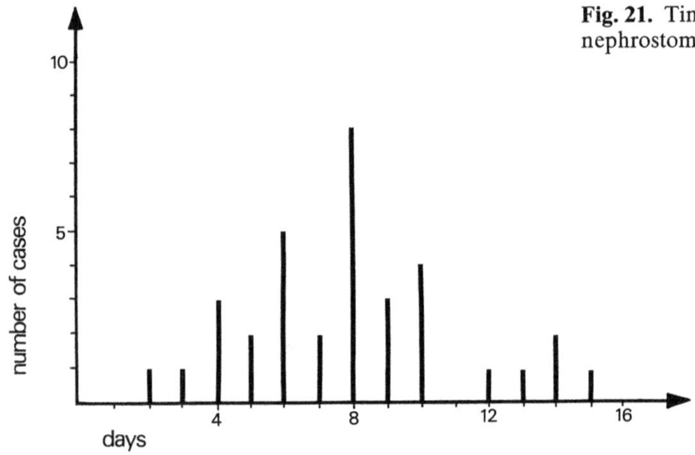

Fig. 21. Time from performance of nephrostomy to full canal dilatation

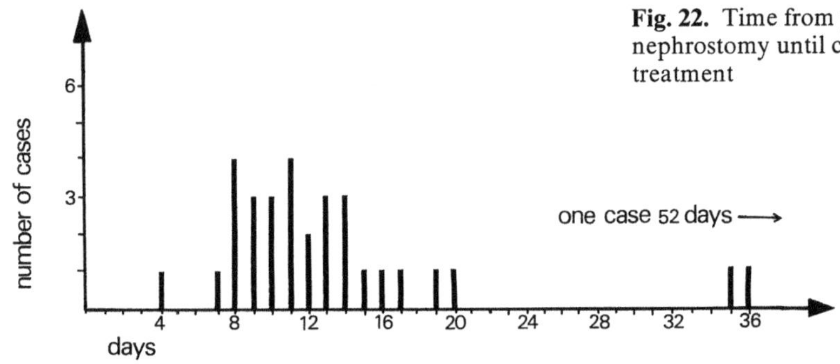

Fig. 22. Time from performance of nephrostomy until completion of treatment

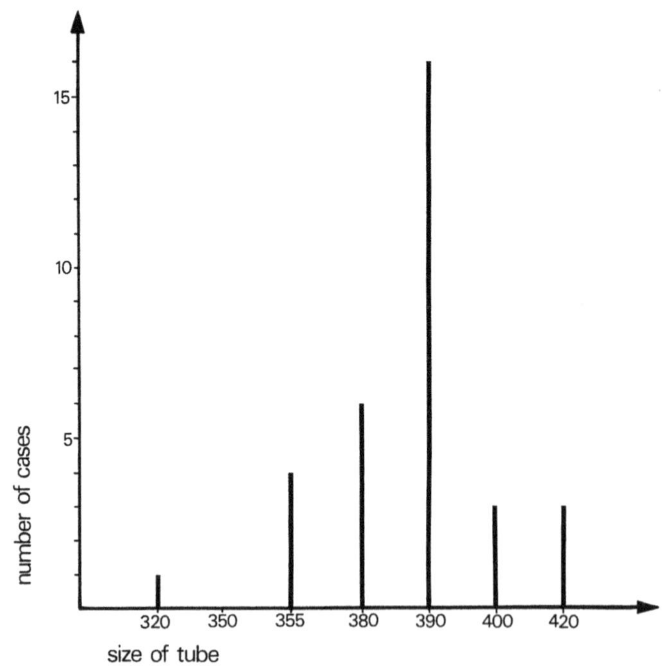

Fig. 23. Maximum tube size used for canal dilatation

Table 1. Success of extraction in relation to position of the stone and operative or percutaneous nephrostomy

	Percutaneous nephrostomy cases		Cases with operative nephrostomy for residual stones	
Stone position	Successful	Failed	Successful	Failed
Calix	11	1	3	4
Renal pelvis	19	1	2	2
Ureter	4	3	0	0
Total	34	5	5	6

not exceed 10–12 mm in diameter (*Hildell* et al. 1980) the present results do not support this suggestion. Nevertheless, we have not generally attempted to remove stones greater than 20 mm in diameter.

The total number of extractions performed are shown in Fig. 26. In most cases the stones were delivered either on the first day or at the second attempt after a delay of 1–3 days. In two cases it was thought wise, however, to wait 14 days to see whether the stubborn calculus would pass down the ureter spontaneously.

The instruments used for extraction or attempted extraction of more than 50 calculi were: Dormia stone basket for 19, extraction forceps for 10 and a combination of forceps and Dormia basket for the remaining 21.

Of the 50 calculi, 16 (32%) broke up in the renal pelvis or canal during the extraction attempt. Six calculi present within a calyx resisted extraction and had to be pushed to better position. The needle harpoon technique had to be used before they could be delivered.

The length of the extraction procedure varied. In some cases the whole procedure could be completed within a few minutes but especially with calyceal stones or with stones that fragmented it was much longer. Generally, however, the total fluoroscopy time was seldom more than 60 min. With experience the extraction time could be reduced.

3.1 Complications

Both the performance of percutaneous nephrostomy and dilatation of the canal were free from complications with the exception of one patient in whom a 320 dilator tube was spontaneously expelled soon after insertion. The whole procedure was repeated the following day and the final successful outcome did not suffer from this minor sctback.

Neither have the numerous extractions nor the extraction attempts led to any serious complications. There were two cases of haemorrhage: one patient was found to have a 1 cm long tear in the renal pelvis, causing a moderate haemorrhage which was probably the result of somewhat injudicious manipulations with extracting forceps. Further manipulations were avoided. A Foley catheter was used

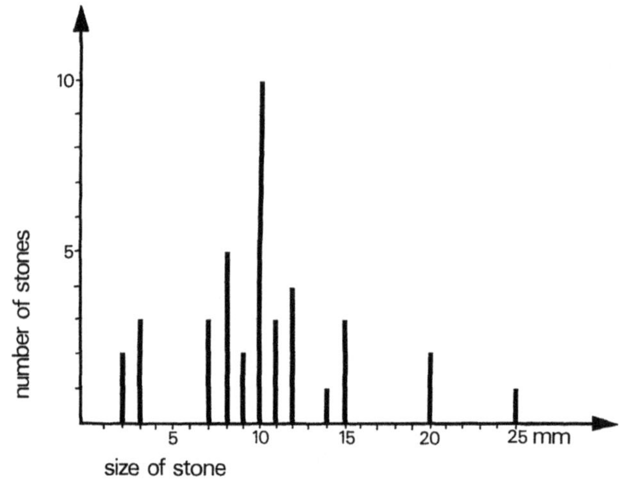

Fig. 24. Size of successfully extracted stones

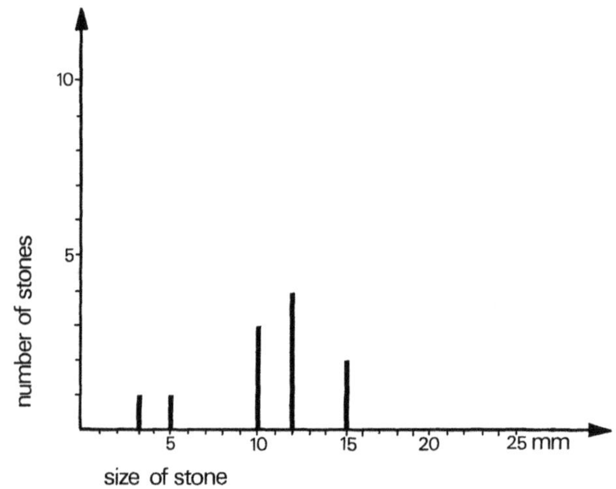

Fig. 25. Size of stones in extraction failures

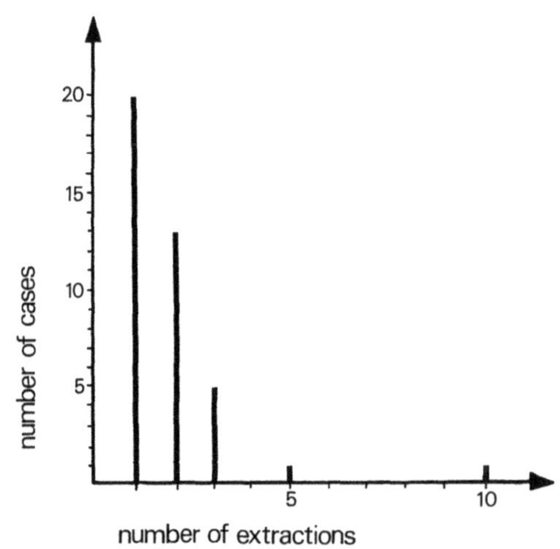

Fig. 26. Number of extraction sessions in each case

to drain and flush the pelvis with saline and the bleeding had ceased by the following day. Bleeding from the dilator tube in one patient was probably due to the tube having perforated a calyx and damaged a small parenchymal vein. The tube had apparently been inserted too far, but even here the bleeding rapidly ceased after the tube was slightly withdrawn. Three patients complained of severe pain during dilatation of the canal. The tubes were of normal type and drained well, and all pain disappeared upon withdrawal. These three patients required the aid of powerful intermittent analgesics during dilatation. The degree of sensitivity of the renal pelvis seems to show considerable individual variation but tends to diminish with age. All patients were given antibiotics prophylactically during their stay in hospital which may explain the lack of infection. Repeated attempts at stone extraction failed in five patients who later underwent open surgery. Additional operative difficulties which could be blamed on the previous nephrostomy or attempts at calculus extraction were not encountered. Even open surgery failed to render three of these patients free from calculi.

Careful follow-up control does not indicate that patients after percutaneous pyelolithotomy are likely to develop subsequent complications such as diminished renal function, arterio-venous fistulae, strictures, hypertension or an increased tendency to recurrent stones.

4 Discussion

Because the technique described did not result in any serious complications and the proportion of stones successfully extracted compared favourably with other more conventional methods, percutaneous pyelolithotomy seems a promising new approach to the treatment of selected cases of renal calculi. Previous reports are too few and the number of cases not numerous enough to evaluate techniques and results.

It is unlikely that any substantial modification in pyelonephrostomy technique is required, although it may be possible to reduce the number of dilatations if special dilators become available. This would, however, save very little time as at least a week must pass before the canal wall is rigid enough to allow an attempt at calculus extraction.

More suitable extraction instruments could certainly be developed, but the cost would be high. Those instruments commonly found in departments of surgery/urology have been used in this study.

If the stone can be moved into the renal pelvis there is usually no difficulty in catching and extracting it, provided that the disparity between the size of the stone and the diameter of the canal is not too great.

Although the difference has been as large as 10 mm even in successful cases (Fig. 23), extraction through the canal is more difficult and too marked a disparity is not recommended.

In the majority of cases the canal is ready for instrumentation after 8 days and the stone removed after 10–12 days. The patient can be discharged 17 days after the

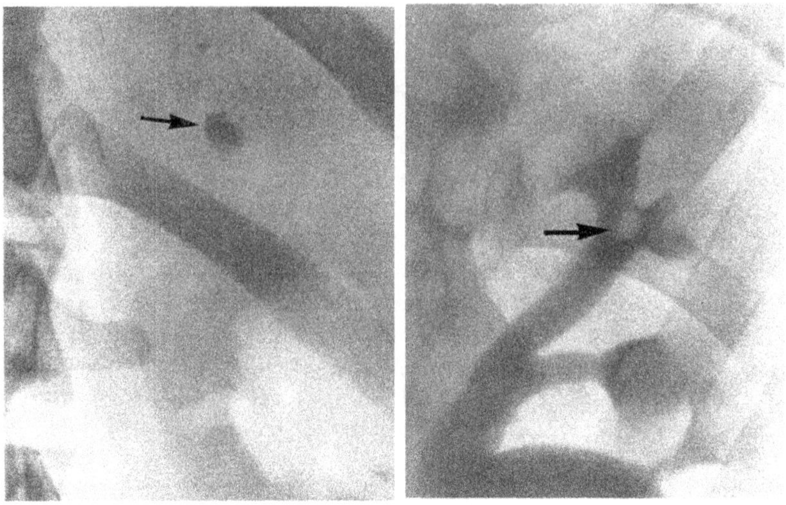

a b

Fig. 27 a, b. Patient who suffered severe pain from a small calyx calculus but whose symptoms completely disappeared following its removal. **a** Plain film with calculus clearly visible (*arrow*); **b** urography with stone appearing as a contrast defect (*arrow*)

performance of percutaneous nephrostomy. It is unlikely that these periods can be substantially shortened and the total length of hospital stay was about the same as that of a normal operation. The advantage of percutaneous pyelolithotomy is, therefore, not in shortening hospitalisation but in treating cases where normal operation is deemed impossible, inopportune or risky. Although an occasional patient could return home much sooner, this is balanced against those who required a considerably longer stay because of extraction difficulties. Length of hospitalisation should not to be compared with that for patients undergoing a primary "simple" stone operation, however, as the patients presented here were all difficult cases who would have required a much longer stay in hospital, and perhaps further surgery before possible success.

Many patients who had previously undergone surgery were asked their opinion of the two methods. Most considered percutaneous pyelolithotomy to be "easier." As mentioned previously, however, a few patients found canal dilatation and stone extraction painful. It was not unusual that more than one extraction session was required. Failure may depend on bleeding or difficulties in negotiating the canal with an instrument. A repeated attempt can be made using a slightly different technique, e.g. with the patient supine instead of prone or with a different extraction instrument.

With normal surgical technique it is often difficult to guarantee complete removal of all small calculi or fragments which may hide in unrecognized recesses, whereas even these stones are often seen and can be extracted when the whole kidney can be inspected on a television screen.

Ease of extraction is related to stone diameter. Calculi greater than 20 mm are not suitable for percutaneous nephrolithotomy because of the excessive degree of

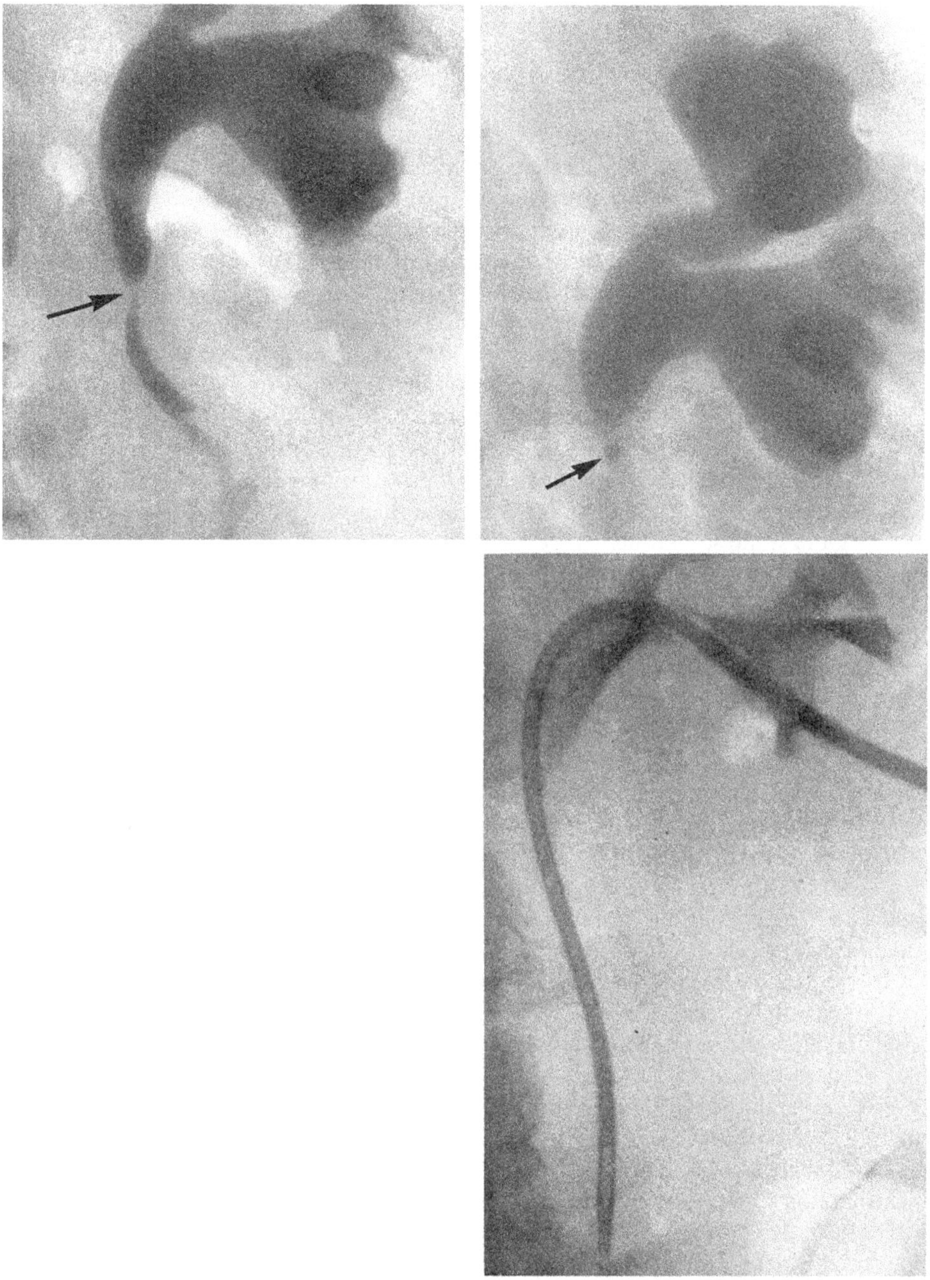

a b c

Fig. 28a–c. A 3×3 mm pelvic stone in a patient with a high postoperative ureteric stricture and mild hydronephrosis. The stone caused intermittent obstruction with acute attacks of pain. After percutaneous stone extraction, the stricture was dilated by a radiopaque catheter (OD = 2.8) and left in position with the tip at the LV level for 14 days. Follow-up 1 year later shows a sustained effect of dilatation and a well-functioning kidney. **a** Urography taken prior to the stone formation (stricture = *arrow*). **b** Urography showing a stone above the stricture (*arrow*) and mild hydronephrosis. **c** A catheter is passed through the stricture and left as a dilator for 14 days canal dilatation which would be required. Furthermore, these large stones seldom cause any operative difficulties even in the presence of fibrosis after previous surgery. Calculi less than 20 mm in diameter are usually easily extracted, although the very small stones can sometimes be difficult to locate and catch. Our best results have been with stones in the renal pelvis or a calyx when the nephrostomy was performed percutaneously. Poor results mainly seem related to kidneys that have been recently operated on with attempts via a peroperatively inserted nephrostomy tube. Under these circumstances the stones tend to adhere to the calyces or pelvic wall. This could be verified at subsequent surgery. Moreover, the position of the peroperatively inserted tube is not always ideal for extraction of a retained stone. It is usually easier in these cases to perform a new nephrostomy percutaneously than to attempt extraction via the unsuitable tube.

Most urologists recognize that some ureteric stones are notoriously difficult to extract. During attempts to remove these stones by percutaneous pyelolithotomy, possible reasons for these difficulties became apparent. Oedema of the ureteric wall grasping the stone sometimes made passage of a Dormia basket impossible, or even if the basket could be manoeuvered past the stone, it could not be opened sufficiently. Failure to deliver a successfully caught stone was a third difficulty. Withdrawal of the Dormia basket sometimes did not move the stone in the ureter, but accomplished a movement of the stone and ureter – the concertina effect. Undue tension on the instrument can in this situation result in a ureteric rupture.

It may seem surprising that many of the successfully removed calculi were situated within a calyx in such a position that they were not particularly amenable to extraction. Success did not depend on a direct approach and extraction, but moving the stone into the renal pelvis by various ingenious manoeuvres. From this position extraction presented no great difficulty.

About one-third of all calculi broke up during extraction, some in the renal pelvis and some while being eased through the canal. Removal of these small fragments was often time consuming.

In six patients with solitary small stones peripherally in a calyx, extraction was performed solely because of severe pain. None of these cases showed diminished renal function or drainage and in all patients pain was relieved as soon as the stone had been extracted. It, therefore, seems that even small stationary stones can give severe pain, although they do not cause urinary stasis. The reason for this is obscure but probably depends on individual variation in sensitivity of the renal pelvis, which may also explain why some patients seemed totally unaffected during manipulation of the stone via the tube, while others required strong analgesics. The cases illustrated in Figs. 9 and 27 are good examples of how small calyceal stones may cause severe pain which can be completely eliminated after extraction.

These small stones can be difficult to locate during open surgery and percutaneous pyelolithotomy should therefore be the method of choice even in these "virgin" cases.

A 3×3 mm renal pelvic stone in a patient with a high postoperative ureteric stricture and mild hydronephrosis is of a special interest. In those situations, extraction of a stone may be combined with dilatation of the stricture as shown in Fig. 28. This case demonstrates the versatility of percutaneous nephrostomy for intrarenal manipulation. Two additional patients, not included in the present material, have subsequently been treated with a similar stricture dilatation technique.

Percutaneous pyelolithotomy ought not to be more trying for the patient than routine open surgery and perhaps even less so. The present investigation was only associated with a few minor complications of which the most alarming, bleeding, always ceased spontaneously. More and wider trials are, however, perhaps required before the place of percutaneous pyelolithotomy within the therapeutic arsenal can be finally assessed.

In order to gain experience in overcoming the various difficulties encountered and to become accustomed to the technique, all percutaneous nephrostomies, canal dilatation and stone extraction attempts have been performed by the same operator (I.F.). It is difficult to judge, therefore, whether similar results could be attained by others. Nevertheless, in our opinion an operator versed in the use of diagnostic radiology and with wide experience of angiography and percutaneous nephrostomy ought to have similar success with percutaneous pyelolithotomy as presented above.

5 Summary

Extraction of renal calculi via a nephrostomy canal was performed in 39 patients with a total of 50 calculi ranging from 3 to 22 mm in diameter. The method used and results obtained are described in detail. The degree of success is probably better than could be obtained with surgical removal in these difficult cases. Following percutaneous nephrostomy, stones lying in the renal pelvis or a calyx could invariably be extracted, but success was limited to 50% for those in the upper ureter. When a nephrostomy was performed at completion of an unsuccessful operation, only half of the residual stones could be removed via the poorly positioned canal. No serious complications have been encountered and the method described can be recommended for patients considered to be poor operative risks of those with difficult, recurrent or residual stones. Hospitalisation was not prolonged and there was less discomfort for the patient.

Since this paper has got into press the total number of cases is now 62 and the results are still very good.

References

Almgård LE, Fernström I (1974) Percutaneous nephropyelostomy. Acta Radiol [Diag] (Stockh) 15:288–294

Andersson L, Fernström I, Leopold GR, Schlegel JU, Telner LB (1977) Radionuclides in urology. Urological ultrasonography. Percutaneous puncture nephrostomy. Diagn Radiol 163–169

Bissada NK, Meacham KR, Redman JF (1974) Nephrostoscopy with removal of renal pelvic calculi. J Urol 112:414–415

Boycel WH (1978) Year book of urology. Yearbook Med Pub, Chicago London 49–50

Brantley RG, Shirley SW (1974) U-tube nephrostomy: an aid in the postoperative removal of retained renal stones. J Urol 111:7–8

Burhenne HJ (1973) Nonoperative retained billary tract stone extraction: a new roentgenolic technique. Am J Roentgenol 177:388–399

Fernström I, Johansson B (1976) Percutaneous pyelolithotomy. A new extraction technique. Scand J Urol Nephrol 10:257–259

Fernström I, Johansson B (to be published) Percutaneous pyelolithotomy. Five years experience. Scand J Urol Nephrol

Hellsten S, Frank B, Hildell J (1980) Percutaneous pyelolithotomy. Case report and technical comments. Eur Urol 6:50–52

Hildell J, Aspelin P, Sigfússon B (1980) Percutaneous nephrostomy. Aspects on clinical application. Acta Radiologica [Diagn] (Stockh) 21:485–490

Karamcheti A, O'Donnell WF (1977) Percutaneous nephrolithotomy: an innovative extraction technique. J Urol 118:671–672

Palestrant AM, Rad FF, Sacks BA, Klein LA (1980) Postoperative Percutaneous Kidney Stone Extraction. Radiology 134:778–779

Rupel E, Brown R (1941) Nephroscopy with removal of stone following nephrostomy for obstructive calculous anuria. J Urol 46:177–182

Percutaneous Nephropyelostomy and Endo-Urological Manipulations

R. Günther and P. Alken[1]

1 Institut für klinische Strahlenkunde und Urologische Klinik der Universität Mainz, Langenbeckstr. 1, D-6500 Mainz

1 Introduction

After a long period of neglect (*Goodwin* et al. 1955), percutaneous nephropyelostomy (PNS) has gained general acceptance and replaced operative nephrostomy. In addition, the percutaneous approach has led to a number of new diagnostic and therapeutic procedures. The objective of this review is not to give a complete and detailed survey of PNS but rather to report on our technique and results with fine needle nephrostomy and various endo-urological manipulations.

2 Percutaneous Nephropyelostomy (PNS)

Numerous technical variations have been described in the literature (*Barbaric* and *Wood* 1977; *Burnett* et al. 1976; *Fernström* and *Andersson* 1977; *Goodwin* et al. 1955; *Günther* et al. 1977, 1979; *Levy* et al. 1979; *Link* et al. 1979; *Pfister* and *Newhouse* 1979; *Stables* et al. 1978). The principle of our technique is a one-step fine needle puncture with subsequent catheter insertion using the same needle tract (Fig. 1). The fine needle allows several puncture attempts without causing major damage to the kidney. Fluoroscopy permits control during the procedure but the combination of real-time ultrasound puncture and fluoroscopic catheter placement, however, seems to be optimal (*Hutschenreiter* et al. 1979). This approach minimizes radiation exposure and allows PNS to be used in children and even in emergency cases during pregnancy. Computerised tomography guided puncture (*Haaga* et al. 1977) is basically unnecessary.

2.1 Technique

The puncture set consists of a long fine needle (length 21 cm, o.d. 0.7 mm) and a shorter two-part nephrostomy needle (Fig. 1) (length 12 cm, o.d. 1.3 mm). The

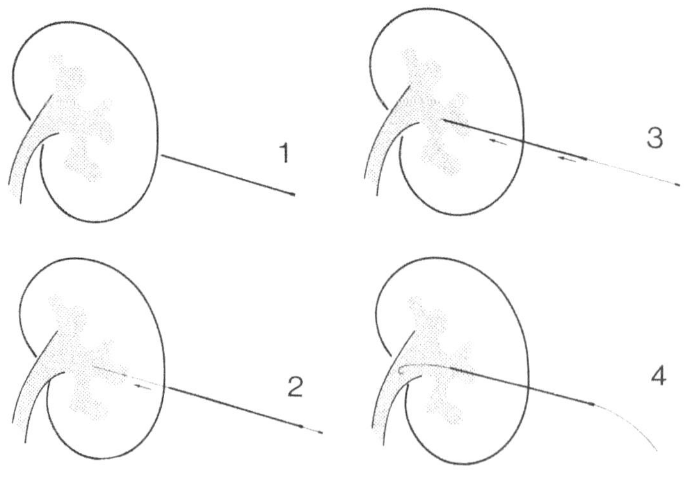

Fig. 1. Scheme for one-step, fine needle puncture for percutaneous nephrostomy

Table 1. Applications of percutaneous nephropyelostomy (PNS)

Diagnostic	Therapeutic
1. Antegrade pyelography	1. Decompression in postrenal obstruction
2. Perfusion pressure studies	2. Diversion in urinary fistulae
3. Assessment of renal functional recovery following decompression	3. Endo-urological manipulations
4. Percutaneous brush biopsy	Antegrade ureteral splinting
5. Percutaneous nephroscopy	Percutaneous catheter extraction
	Percutaneous litholapaxy and stone extraction
	Percutaneous irrigation (stone dissolution, chemotherapy, antibiotics)
	Percutaneous meatotomy
	Percutaneous dilatation of ureteral stenoses
	Transrenal ureteral embolization

Table 2. Therapeutic applications of percutaneous nephropyelostomy in 202 patients

	No.
I. Decompression in postrenal obstruction	
Obstructing calculus	21
Obstructing tumour	18
Ureteral obstruction not secondary to neoplasia (Crohn's disease, retroperitoneal fibrosis, tuberculosis, radiogenic stenosis, postoperative stricture)	22
Ureteropelvic junction obstruction	17
Postoperative obstruction due to oedema following ureteral reimplantation	10
Atresia of the ureter	1
Megaureter	2
Infravesical obstruction due to urethral valves	3
II. External diversion in urinary fistulae or extravasation	9
III. Endo-urological manipulations	
1. Antegrade ureteral splinting	34
2. Percutaneous stone manipulation	33
3. Transrenal catheter extraction	4
4. Transrenal ureteral embolization	28
Total	202

inner stylet used originally is dispensable. Prior intravenous administration of contrast medium opacifies the upper urinary tract.

In non-functioning kidneys the puncture site is chosen with the aid of real-time ultrasound. For children a smaller size puncture set is available (*Günther* and *Alken* 1979).

Under local anaesthesia in a prone position the short two-part nephrostomy needle is pushed through the musculature and fascia to the perirenal space from the posterolateral lumbar region (*Goodwin* et al. 1955; *Günther* et al. 1977). Once the perirenal space is reached, the long fine needle is inserted and the kidney is punctured with continuous infiltration of lignocaine until the needle tip is located

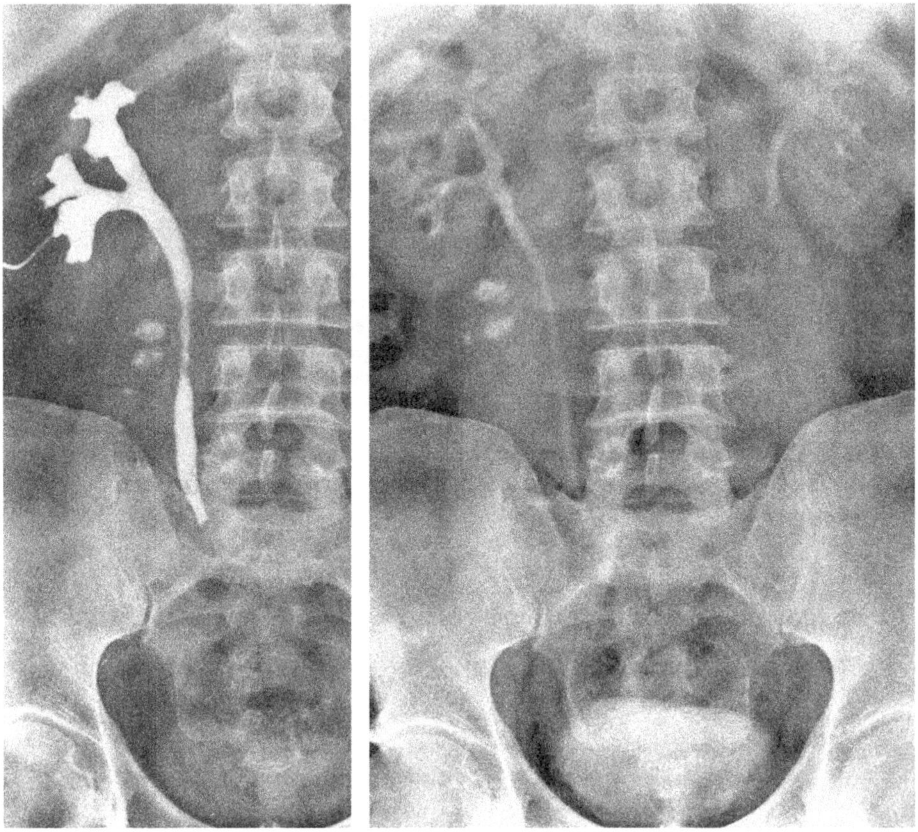

a b

Fig. 2a, b. Percutaneous nephrostomy in ureteral obstruction due to uric acid stones. (Emergency indication: development of septic fever following retrograde pyelogram in an outside hospital). Following decompression the stones passed spontaneously. Normal IVP 2 weeks after PNS

within the renal pelvis or a calyx. Only in non-dilated pyelocalyceal system an additional thin guide wire (o.d. 0.5 mm) is used to fix the needle tip. Subsequently, the fine needle serves as a guide over which the nephrostomy needle can be advanced. In the Seldinger technique a J guide wire (o.d. 0.9 mm) is introduced for catheter placement. A 5 F thin-walled tube provided with several side holes suffices for initial drainage.

If pus or thick fluid must be drained, the tract is further dilated up to 14 F. For long-term drainage silicone tubes are preferred.

2.2 Indications

Percutaneous nephropyelostomy offers a large variety of diagnostic and therapeutic applications (Table 1). Its importance lies mainly in the non-operative management of and therapy for upper urinary tract disease (Table 2). The percutaneous access permits decompression in postrenal obstruction, external urinary diversion in

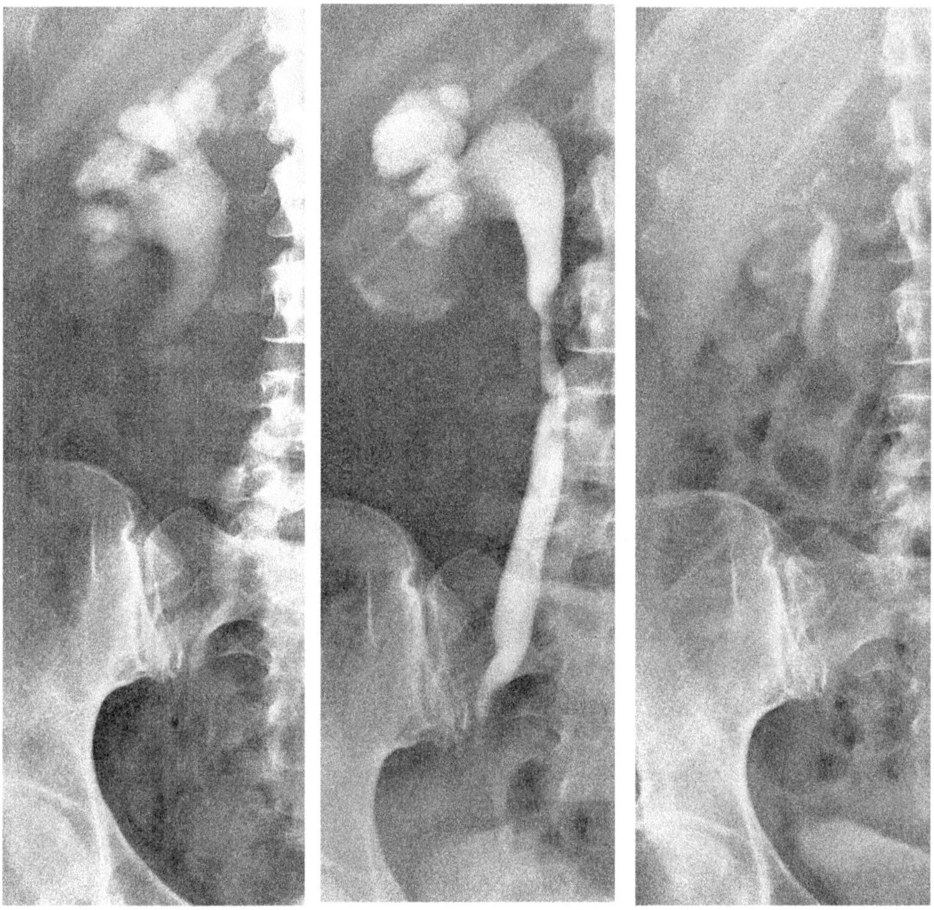

a b, c

Fig. 3a–c. Percutaneous nephrostomy as a temporary measure to preserve renal function during tuberculostatic therapy. **a** IVP showing obstruction of the distal ureter; **b** PNS under tuberculostatic cover; **c** result after resection of the stenotic ureteral segment and reimplantation of the ureter

urinary fistulae and endo-urological manipulations. For practical reasons the indications can be divided in two main groups:

1. *Emergency indications:*
   a) Postrenal obstruction complicated by fever, septicaemia and uraemia (Fig. 2)
   b) Postoperative fistulae causing urinoma
2. *Non-emergency indications:*
   a) Drainage until clarification of the underlying disease
   b) Drainage during chemotherapy or radiotherapy (Fig. 3) (e.g. Hodgkin's disease, Crohn's disease, tuberculosis etc.)
   c) Management of urinary fistulae (Fig. 4)

Originally PNS was developed as an emergency procedure and has adopted the classic indications for operative nephrostomy: postrenal obstruction with infection

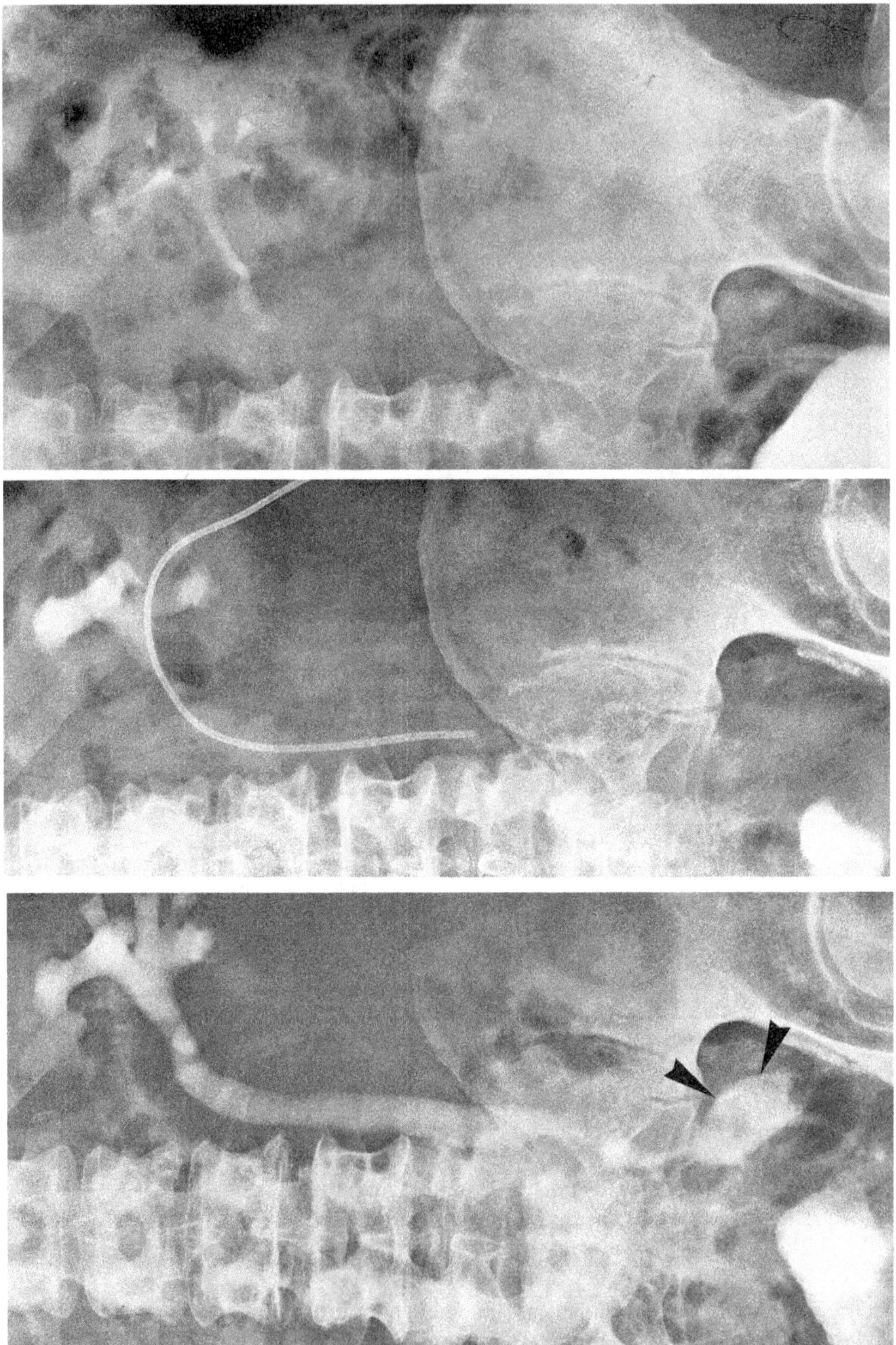

a b c

and uraemia. While uncomplicated obstruction is usually tolerated by the kidney for months, superinfection leads to a rapid loss of renal function and parenchymal destruction, thus requiring urgent decompression. The need for diversion in uraemia due to postrenal obstruction is obvious. The advantages of PNS are convincing: the procedure can be done under local anaesthesia, causes little discomfort to the patient and permits delay of the operation until the patient has recovered and can be operated upon under more favourable circumstances.

Urinary fistulae may develop following urological operations, abdominal surgery, irradiation and trauma. Small fistulae may heal solely by conservative means using external drainage or internal splinting, large fistulae do not dry out. If the patient's clinical condition is acceptable, primary surgery is the method of choice. In widespread tumour disease, however, transrenal ureteral occlusion combined with PNS is recommended (Sect. 6).

2.3 **Results** (Tables 2 and 3)

In 202 patients, 228 percutaneous nephrostomies were performed. In 94 the aim was decompression in postrenal obstruction secondary to various lesions: stones, tumours, obstruction of other origin, postoperative oedema or stricture following reimplantation of the ureter and, in rare cases, infravesical obstruction. Adequate drainage was achieved in all cases. Subsequent operation on two patients whose fever did not subside revealed pyonephrosis with multiple parenchymal abscesses.

In ten patients with inoperable pelvic malignancy the external drainage remained the definitive and permanent solution. The method proved to be most useful in postoperative complications following ureteral surgery (oedema at the anastomosis, leakage) ($n = 19$) (Fig. 4). In one patient with uric acid stone obstruction the calculi passed spontaneously within 2 weeks following decompression (Fig. 2). In seven of nine cases urinary fistulae closed following external drainage.

The puncture success in our series of 228 procedures was 95% (Table 3). In 75% the punctures succeeded within the first three attempts. This is comparable to the results obtained with ultrasound (*Hutschenreiter* et al. 1979).

2.4 Limitations

A prerequisite for PNS is the absence of a coagulopathy. Thrombocyte count should be over 80 000/mm^3 and prothrombin time under 50%. Other contra-indications are severe hypertension and untreated tuberculosis.

Prior to employing PNS, its benefits must be thoroughly evaluated. PNS is most valuable for short-term drainage, while multiple problems, such as tube obstruction, dislocation and discomfort of the outer appliance, may arise in long-term drainage. In addition, there are potential serious complications such as chronic infection, stone formation and progressive renal deterioration. Therefore, long-term

Fig. 4a–c. Percutaneous nephrostomy in urinary fistulae. **a** Extravasation and obstruction in the distal ureter following deep anterior resection of the rectum; **b** external drainage; **c** normal IVP 2 years later

Table 3. Percutaneous nephropyelostomy (PNS); a survey of 228 procedures (202 patients)

Patients (n)	PNS (n)	Successful puncture	Complications
181 adults	198	94%	4.5%
21 children	30	97%	–
	228	95%	4%

Table 4. Percutaneous nephropyelostomy: complications in 228 procedures (202 patients)

	No.
Minor	
Accidental catheter breakage	2
Minor bleeding with blood clots in the renal pelvis	2
Small perirenal haematoma	2
Major	
Septicaemia without sequelae	1
Major bleeding (retroperitoneal haematoma, arterial bleeding 2 weeks after initial placement of the catheter)	2
Total	9

Table 5. Operative nephropyelostomy: complications in 167 patients

	No.
Postoperative bleeding (requiring reintervention in six and nephrectomy in three patients)	12
Lesion of the pleura	9
Lesion of the peritoneum	3
Lesion of the renal vein	1
Lesion of the ureter	1
Respiratory insufficiency	3
Cardiac arrest	1
Diabetic coma	3
Total	33
Deaths due to:	
Uraemia	2
Sepsis	3
Protracted shock	2
Cardiac decompensation	2
Total	9

nephrostomy drainage should be avoided if at all possible. If PNS remains the sole treatment, it may happen that in isolated cases another coexisting renal disease will be overlooked as was the case with one of our patients: after unsuccessful percutaneous stone manipulation only subsequent operation disclosed a small renal cell carcinoma.

Because of its simplicity the method may be used with too great a frequency, especially in far-advanced pelvic malignant disease. PNS should not prolong suffering unnecessarily. Thus, urinary diversion is unjustifiable in cases with intractable pains and poor condition in terminal cancer (*Fallon* et al. 1980; *Holden* et al. 1979; *Sharer* et al. 1978).

2.5 Complications

Complications were encountered in 9 of 228 procedures (4%; tables 3 and 4). Among them were three major complications: One patient developed septicaemia without sequelae. Bleeding in a second patient led to a large retroperitoneal haematoma which was found at surgery 3 days after unsuccessful catheter positioning. In this case, the kidney was removed because of septicaemia. In a third, major haemorrhage due to erosion of an artery occurred after removal of the catheter 2 weeks after initial placement and could be stopped by reinsertion of a larger tube. Transient haematuria was not regarded as a complication. In 15 patients catheter displacement could be corrected be reinsertion without repuncture. Longterm drainage for more than 1 year was complicated by stone formation in two patients.

The rate of major complications according to the literature is 4% (*Stables* et al. 1978). Only one death due to bleeding was observed by *Fernström* and *Andersson* (1978). In a follow-up study of 167 patients undergoing operative nephrostomy at our hospital the complication rate amounted to 25.1% including nine deaths (5.4%) (Table 5). *Gonzales-Serva* et al. (1977) reported an operative mortality rate of 6%. Although the operative and percutaneous series are not completely comparable because of different selection of patients there is no doubt that considering only emergency cases, which are comparable in both groups, the operative nephrostomy is more risky than the percutaneous approach.

3 Antegrade Ureteral Splinting/Stenting

Ureteral splint placement via the percutaneous nephrostomy tract offers an alternative to the retrograde cystoscopic approach (*Bigongiari* et al. 1979; *Finney* 1978; *Goldin* 1977; *Günther* and *Alken* 1980; *Kearney* et al. 1979, *Lang* 1981; *Mazer* et al. 1979; *Pfister* and *Newhouse* 1979). In contrast to nephrostomy drainage, the ureteral splint permits natural urine passage and thus avoids external appliances. There are several possibilities for splint placement:

1. Indwelling splint
2. Percutaneous splint with subcutaneous implantation
3. Percutaneous splint with fixation at the skin

Indwelling splints and splints with subcutaneous fixation of the proximal occluded end are preferable because of their lower infection rate. The disadvantage of the indwelling splint is that it is not accessible to irrigation, and, in case of obstruction, necessitates cystoscopic or transrenal extraction.

3.1 Technique

3.1.1 Indwelling Splint

Following PNS, ureteral splinting is performed after an interval of 2–3 days in order to avoid blood clot obstruction. The procdure is carried out under local anaesthesia in a right or left oblique supine position. After introduction of a J guide wire (o.d. 1.0 mm) the nephrostomy catheter is exchanged for a 5 F polythene catheter. The stenotic area is gently probed and finally passed. Leaving the guide in place with the tip in the bladder the catheter is withdrawn. The length of the splint is tailored to the length of the ureter. With the aid of a 'pusher' the splint provided with multiple side holes is advanced down the ureter until the distal end is in the bladder and the proximal end is in the pyelocalyceal system (Fig. 5). The critical point is that the indwelling splint is stuck in the stricture without being accessible any more from outside. Therefore, the splint must not be too short. After removal of the pusher a 5 F nephrostomy tube is left in place for 2 days, permitting direct access to the kidney in case of splint obstruction. Buckling of the splint during insertion indicates that the forward force applied from outside does not suffice to pass the stenosis. Nevertheless, the procedure can be accomplished successfully with cystoscopic aid by grasping and straightening the guide wire. Thus, the force applied is better transferred to the tip of the splint. If the manoeuvre fails from above, the guide wire is brought out the urethra transcystoscopically and retrograde splinting is performed.

3.1.2 Percutaneous Splint with Extrarenal Fixation

Probing of the ureter is done as described above. For splinting a longer piece of catheter provided with multiple side holes for drainage of the urinary tract is used. The proximal occluded end is fixed either subcutaneously or at the skin with a monofil thread (Prolene).
Distinctive aids in negotiating ureteral kinks and stenoses are:

1. J guide with movable core or torque control
2. Steerable catheter (Medi-Tech)
3. Coaxial catheter system [7 F thin-walled polytetrafluoroethylene (Teflon) catheter combined with a 5 F polyethylene catheter].
4. Sturdy Teflon introducer (10 F, 12 F).
5. Grüntzig balloon catheter.

3.1.3 Splint Material

In the selection of splint material the following physical and biological properties are essential: good biocompatibility, flexibility, stability, low tendency towards incrustation, radiopacity and easy insertion over the guide. Polyethylene and polyvinyl

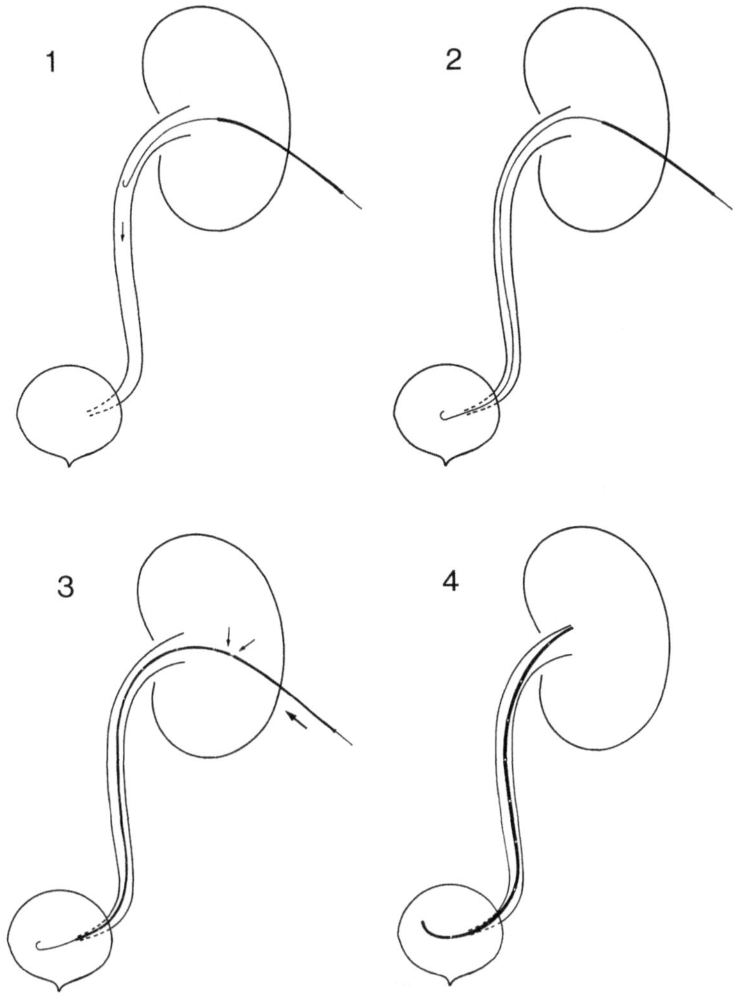

Fig. 5. Scheme for antegrade ureteral splinting (indwelling splint)

chloride (PVC) have a high tendency towards incrustation, but a low friction coefficient. Incrustation is less pronounced with polyurethane and even less with Teflon (*Maar* et al. 1977). Silicone splints are most suitable from the standpoint of biocompatibility (*Weißbach* et al. 1979; *Zimskid* et al. 1967). Its high friction coefficient, however, prevents an easy insertion. A coaxial system (outer silicone catheter, inner 5 F polythene catheter lubricated with silicone spray) proved helpful.

For short-term internal diversion we usually use a 6 F polythene splint or a 8 F PVC splint. Pig-tail configuration, double J-splint or Gibbon's splint may prevent migration or dislocation. For long-term drainage silicone splints are recommended if insertion is technically possible, otherwise Teflon or polyurethane splints are advisable.

Table 6. Indications for antegrade ureteral splinting [a]

I. Pre-operative decompression and intra-operative assistance		
Retroperitoneal fibrosis, ureterolysis with intraperitoneal placement of the ureter		1
II. Operative complications		
Accidental ligation of the ureter		1
III. Postoperative complications		16
Obstruction following:		
Ureterolysis	1	
Nephropyelolithotomy	3	
Colon conduit diversion	4	
Psoas-hitch-plasty	1	
Boari-plasty	2	
Cohen-antireflux-plasty	2	
Obstruction and extravasation following:		
Ureterolysis	1	
Tumour resection in solitary kidney	1	
Pyelolithotomy	1	
IV. Strictures		3
Radiogenic	1	
Following ureterotomy	1	
Following transuretero-ureterocutaneostomy	1	
V. Tumour obstruction		5
Inoperable prostate cancer	2	
Inoperable bladder cancer	1	
Recurrent rectum cancer	1	
Inoperable stomach cancer (metastases)	1	

[a] 26 patients with successful splinting: temporary = 20; permanent = 6

Table 7. Final outcome in 26 patients with antegrade ureteral splinting

Groups I, II, III. (pre-operative, postoperative diversion; n = 18)	
Free urinary flow	4
Urinary leakage closed, no obstruction	3
Moderate persistent obstruction	2
Conversion to external drainage	1
Loop ureterocutaneostomy	1
Colon-conduit diversion	1
Nephrectomy	4
Unknown	2
Group IV (strictures) (n = 3)	
Nephrectomy	1
Moderate persistent obstruction	1
Permanent internal splinting	1
Group V (tumour obstruction) (n = 5)	
Death after 2, 4 and 11 months	3
Conversion to external drainage	1
Unknown	1

In one patient a 7 F thin-walled Teflon splint was used with excellent success for a period of 6 months. After removal there were no macroscopic changes in the splint, nor was there incrustation or obstruction.

3.2 Indications

Indications for ureteral splinting are (Table 6):

1. Ureteral obstruction
   a) Postoperative oedema following ureteral surgery
   b) Pelvic malignancy
2. Management of ureteral fistulae

Antegrade ureteral splinting proved particularly effective in postoperative complications with oedema at the anastomosis following reimplantation of the ureter. In contrast to external nephrostomy drainage the splint keeps the anastomosis patent and wet. Nevertheless operative success in all cases cannot be guaranteed using this approach (Table 7). Small postoperative or post-traumatic urinary fistulae may respond very well (*Lang* 1981). Strictures (postoperative late complications) may hardly be influenced even with previous additional balloon dilatation. In tumour obstruction the same limitations as for PNS are valid. In long-term drainage indwelling splinting is preferable to nephrostomy drainage.

3.3 **Results** (Tables 6 and 7)

Antegrade ureteral splinting was attempted in 34 patients and succeeded in 26. In complete obstruction catheterization usually failed. 20 patients had an indwelling splint, 6 a percutaneous splint with external fixation (5 at the skin, 1 subcutaneously).

In three patients insertion of the splint could be achieved only with the aid of cystoscopy. Splint diversion lasted between 1 week and 12 months; it was temporary in 20 patients and permanent in 6. The majority of patients had postoperative complications following upper urinary tract surgery (17 of 26 patients) (Table 6). During a pre-operative decompression in retroperitoneal fibrosis the ureter was splinted, thus allowing better operative identification of the ureter for ureterolysis and intraperitoneal placement.

In one patient with accidental ureteral ligation splinting was the sole form of treatment and the intravenous pyelogram (IVP) normalized within two months (Table 7 and Fig. 6). In 9 of 18 patients with temporary internal diversion the operative and postoperative complications could be managed with perfect results in 7, and improvement of obstruction in 2 (Table 7). In 4 instances nephrectomy had to be performed.

The outcome in fibrotic ureteral strictures were less encouraging: persistent obstruction, permanent internal splinting and nephrectomy were the results.

In tumour obstruction no more than palliation was expected (Fig. 7).

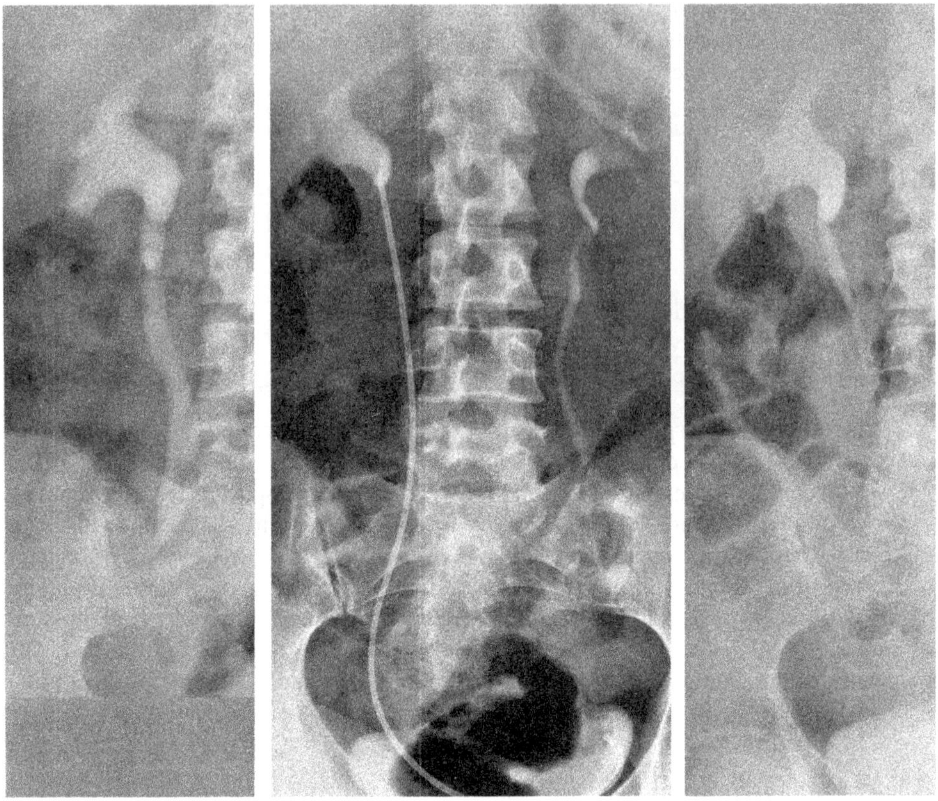

a b, c

Fig. 6a–c. Antegrade indwelling splinting for management of accidental ligation of the ureter during hysterectomy. **a** IVP; **b** indwelling splint; **c** normalization of the IVP following cystoscopic removal of the splint

3.4 Complications (Table 8)

In total we observed 14 complications mainly due to dislocation, incrustation, bending and insufficient drainage. In one patient a perirenal haematoma was found at subsequent surgery. Apart from splint problems infection is not uncommon especially in long-term drainage.

Table 8. Complications of antegrade ureteral splinting in 26 patients

	No.
Splint displacement	5
Splint obstruction (after 3 d, 3 and 4 wks, 1 mo)	4
Splint incrustation (after 3 and 12 mos)	2
Splint bending	1
Insufficient internal drainage	1
Perirenal haematoma	1
Total	14

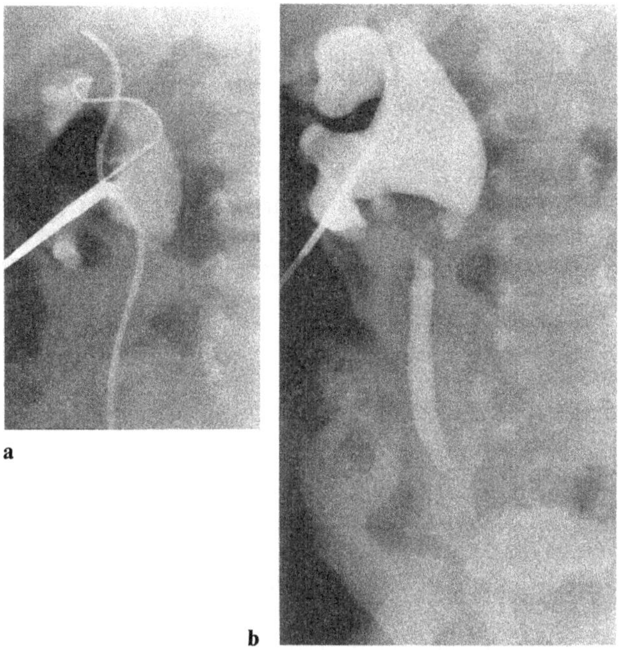

a b

Fig. 8a, b. Percutaneous removal of an obstructed indwelling splint using forceps

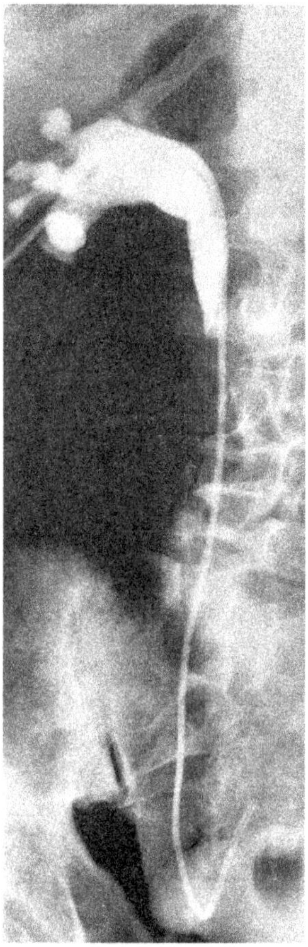

Fig. 7. Percutaneous ureteral splinting in metastasizing prostate cancer; good general condition of the patient

4 Percutaneous Catheter Extraction

4.1 Technique

The procedure is carried out through the previously dilated nephrostomy channel. A sturdy 9 F Teflon catheter (length 20 cm) with a bend at the tip is inserted into the renal pelvis using a J guide wire. A Dormia stone basket or foreign body grasping forceps serve to extract the catheter (Fig. 8). The grasping forceps must be handled very cautiously. Since they are not steerable, slight rotation of the preformed tip of the catheter permits localization and grasping of the retained catheter.

Following extraction, PNS is re-established. As an added precaution during manipulation, the nephrostomy channel is secured by a guide wire (Fig. 8).

4.2 Indications

One of the complications of PNS or antegrade internal splinting is catheter obstruction or tearing. The latter usually occurs if unsuitable material is used. If cystoscopical removal of these catheter fragments or splints fails, percutaneous access is the method of choice.

4.3 Results

Percutaneous extraction via the nephrostomy tract was attempted in four patients and succeeded in three. A broken nephrostomy tube was found in three patients and in one an obstructed indwelling splint. No complications have been encountered as a consequence of the manipulations.

5 Percutaneous Stone Manipulations [1]

Stones in the upper urinary tract are accessible to percutaneous manipulations via the nephrostomy tract. Displacement, dissolution, extraction or fragmentation by forceps are well known (*Fernström* and *Andersson* 1977; *Fernström* and *Johansson* 1976; *Karamcheti* and *O'Donnel* 1977; *Mulvaney* 1960; *Pfister* and *Newhouse* 1979; *Rupel* and *Brown* 1941; *Smith* et al. 1979a; *Suby* and *Albright* 1943; *Weiss* et al. 1976); fragmentation by ultrasound was only recently applied in a larger series (*Alken* et al. 1981).

5.1 Technique

5.1.1 Dissolution

Various fluids are currently used for stone dissolution: urate calculi are dissolved by alkalinizing solutions which are also used in combination with N-actylcysteine for cystine calculi. Organic acids (e.g. hemiacidrin) are suitable for stones containing struvite and apatite. The stone is irrigated through a 6 F–8 F catheter at a flow rate of 100 ml/h. We adhere to the following guidelines: the patient must be afebrile, the urine sterile and the nephrostogram must demonstrate free flow without extravasation.

An internal splint or double nephrostomy is helpful if distal ureteral obstruction is present. Perfusion is immediatly discontinued at the first sign of fever or back pain. Creatinine and electrolyte determinations are performed every day. Depending on the size and site of the stone dissolution may last 10–30 days.

5.1.2 Extraction

Small stones may be removed from the renal pelvis or the proximal ureter with the aid of a Dormia stone basket, a snare or a pair of Randall forceps. This requires previous dilatation of the nephrostomy tract up to 14 F–20 F.

---

1 Section by *P. Alken*

5.1.3 Ultrasound Fragmentation

Large stones can be fragmented by ultrasound ("litholapaxy or disintegration") via the nephrostomy tract. For this purpose the tract is successively dilated with a set of specially designed metal dilators up to 26 F within 1 week. The final 26 F catheter is left in place for 4–5 days. Afterwards the ultrasound probe[1] is inserted under endoscopic control and fragmentation carried out using a frequency of 20 KHz. The procedure is done under local or peridural anaesthesia.

5.2 Indications

The procedure is especially helpful for poor risk patients or for those with multiple previous stone operations, as multiple operative interventions increase the risk of kidney loss.

The decision whether a stone should by dissolved, extracted or fragmented, depends on its size and composition. Our policy is: small stones are extracted, large stones are disintegrated by ultrasound.

Smaller stones in the pelvis are accessible to extraction by Randall forceps. Stones in the upper third of the ureter may be removed by a snare or Dormia stone basket, although the ultrasound probe can also be directed into the dilated ureter. Mechanical fragmentation by ultrasound is suitable for large stones and even staghorn calculi irrespective of their composition. Dilatation of the pyelocalyceal system is not a prerequisite.

Dissolution is used in patients with cystine calculi, which are readily dissolvable. Urate stones are usually dissolved by the peroral adminstration of drugs. Direct irrigation is only applied if the stone has led to obstruction and septicemia. Under these circumstances PNS is performed for decompression and subsequently serves as an access for irrigation.

If earlier stone analysis or infection of the urine with alkalinizing bacteria are indicative of struvite or calcium carbonate apatite stones, dissolution by irrigation with organic acids may be performed for a reasonable period of time.

5.3 **Results** (Tables 9 and 10)

A total number of 47 patients (49 renal units) had stone manipulation and in 33 instances percutaneous nephrostomy was used. Forty-six patients presented with stones in the renal pelvis. In one case additional ureteral stones were present (Fig. 9). Manipulations included dissolution in 9, extraction in 16 and fragmentation by ultrasound in 19. The hospital stay averaged 30 days. In five patients percutaneous technique failed and the stones had to be removed operatively. In two patients small residual stones were observed following fragmentation.

The higher percentage of residual stones in the group of surgical nephrostomies (Table 10) was due to the fact that these were cases where long-term drainage was

1 K. Storz KG, D-7200 Tuttlingen

Table 9. Percutaneous stone manipulation using different techniques in 47 patients (49 kidneys)

Approach		Technique	
Operative nephropyelostomy ($n = 16$)	Stone	Ultrasound litholapaxy	($n = 19$)
		Extraction	($n = 16$)
Percutaneous nephropyelostomy ($n = 33$)		Chemolysis	($n = 9$)
		Unsuccessful	($n = 5$)

Table 10. Success of percutaneous stone manipulations in 47 patients (49 kidneys)

	Manipulations	
	Via percutaneous nephropyelostomy	Via operative nephropyelostomy
Free from stones	26	8
Residual stones	2	8
Unsuccessful [a]	5	–

[a] Stone manipulation was unsuccessful in five patients who required subsequent surgery

complicated by stone development. The primary aim of the manoeuvre was to remove the obstructing pelvic stone and not to completely clear the kidney of every calyceal stone. The high success rate of this method following a primary percutaneous approach can be attributed to the free choice of routes for optimal access to the stone.

5.4 Complications

In two patients bleeding occured during extraction of a stone through the inadequately dilated nephrostomy channel. In one patient pooling of fluid during ultrasound disintegration was observed. These complications were managed conservatively.

6 Transrenal Ureteral Occlusion

Watertight closure of the ureter is the aim of transrenal ureteral embolization. As early as 1911 Kawasoye advised tying a knot the leaking ureter to stop urinary flow (*Murphy* 1972). Despite technical progress and sophisticated operative interventions urinary leakage remains a problem in a small number of patients up to the present day. This prompted us do develop a non-operative solution to this problem.

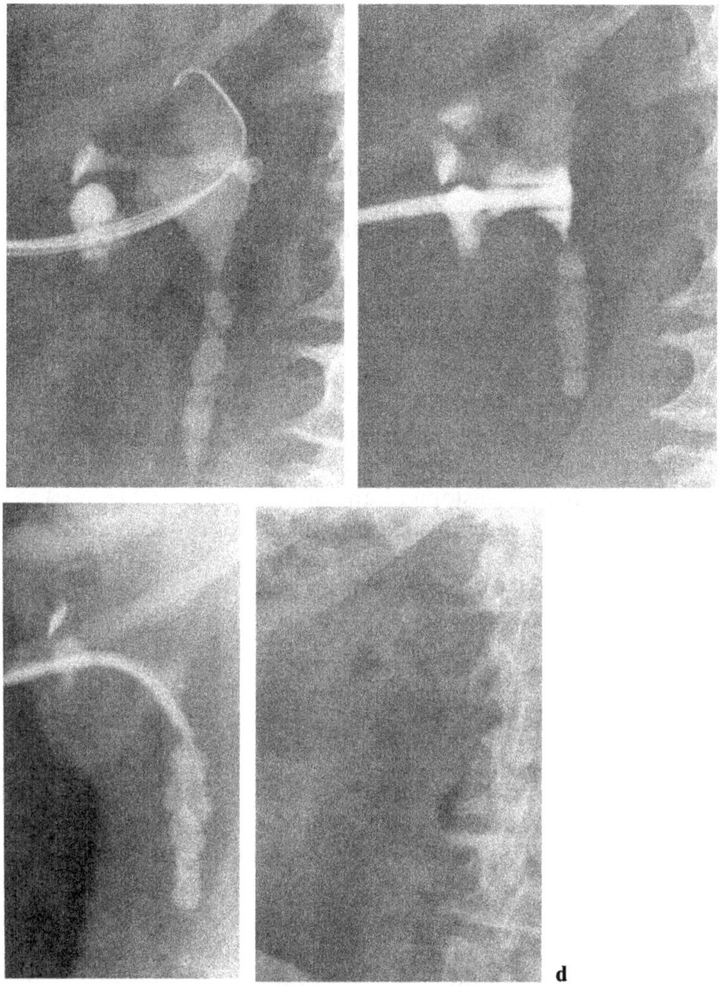

a b c d

Fig. 9 a–d. Percutaneous removal of stones: ultrasound fragmentation of the large stone in the renal pelvis. Ureteral stones were removed using a snare. **a** PNS and dilatation of the nephrostomy tract (26 F); **b** renal pelvis free of stones following ultrasound litholapaxy; **c** percutaneous extraction of the ureteral stones with snare; **d** plain radiograph following completion of the procedure

6.1 Technique

6.1.1 Embolization with Tissue Adhesive (Fig. 10)

Following fine needle PNS the needle tract is dilated with Teflon dilators until a 9 F Teflon introducer (length 30 cm) can be inserted into the proximal ureter with the aid of a J guide. Subsequently, a 5 F Swan-Ganz balloon catheter is advanced into the distal ureter and inflated with 0.2–0.5 ml saline until the ureter is occluded. The embolizing material consists of butyl-2-cyanoacrylate (BC) mixed with lipiodol

(L) and tantalum powder: 1 ml BC+1 ml L+0.3 ml tantalum powder (*Günther* et al. 1980). The mixture is injected under fluoroscopic control. Slight inflation and deflation of the balloon permits determination of polymerization completion. Generally the ureter is filled up to the proximal part. Previous occlusion with a Gianturco coil favours the obstructive effect. After completion of the procedure external urinary drainage is established by nephrostomy.

6.1.2 Occlusion with a Detachable Balloon (Figs. 11 and 12)

This procedure was developed only recently (*Günther* 1981). It requires a 14 F Teflon introducer which is advanced into the proximal part of the ureter. A latex rubber balloon inflatable up to 2 cm in diameter is attached to a 3 F Teflon catheter (length 60 cm) by a fine latex rubber string. This is similar to Debrun's technique for vascular embolization. The outer 5 F Teflon catheter (length 45 cm) improves catheter stability and facilitates balloon detachment. After fluoroscopic placement in the distal portion of the ureter the balloon is slowly filled with a mixture of silicone elastomer[1] and silicone fluid 360 (ratio 1:5) using a tuberculin syringe. Previous addition of catalyst M (2 drops/ml) induces polymerization and tantalum powder (1 g/ml) renders the mixture radiopaque. Depending on the size of the ureter an amount of 0.5–1 ml usually blocks the ureter. Within 15–20 min the mixture polymerizes into a soft rubbery substance and the balloon can be detached. Subsequently external drainage is performed.

6.2 Indications

Transrenal ureteral occlusion is a non-aggressive palliative procedure. General indications are: large urinary fistulae and severe, painful dysuria in advanced pelvic malignancy. In addition, the method has proved useful as an emergency procedure in postoperative complications with large urinary fistulae not manageable by percutaneous drainage alone and is an effective means of preventing formation of abdominal urinomas.

The advantage of ureteral embolization – irrespective of the material used (tissue adhesive, detachable balloon) – is that the ureter is not irreparably lost after removal of the occluding material, but remains amenable to ureteral surgery or operative urinary diversion after the patient has recovered. According to our current experience, the detachable balloon is superior to tissue adhesive.

Severe dysuria responds very well to an interruption of urinary flow, while haematuria is less favourably influenced. Under certain circumstances, total urinary incontinence may be managed by this method as a last resort.

The rationale for non-operative management of urinary fistulae in tumour patients is: in the presence of advanced pelvic malignancy, extensive reconstructive procedures which often require permanent supravesical urinary diversion are not justified. External drainage by percutaneous nephrostomy may suffice for the management of smaller fistulae, but is usually unsuccessful in large leakages. The social and psychological stigma of total urinary incontinence necessitates some

---

1 Dow Corning, D-4000 Düsseldorf

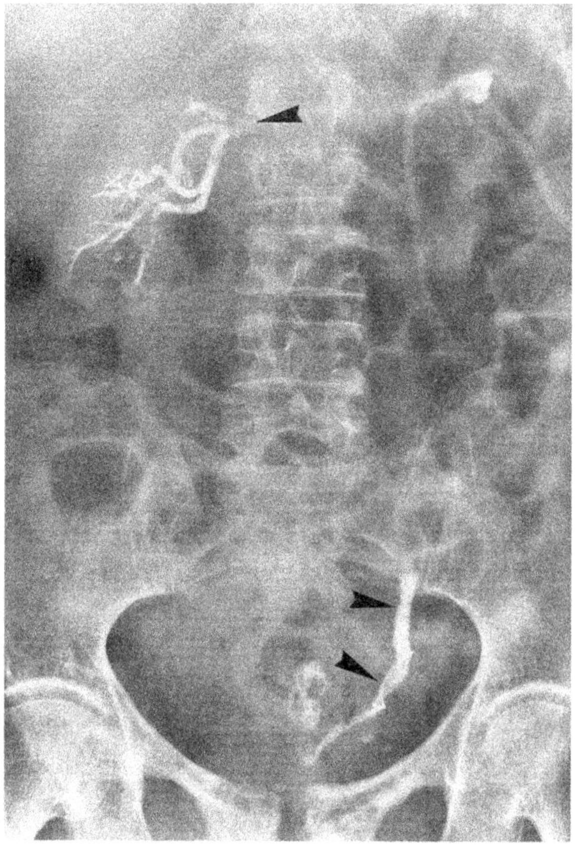

Fig. 10. Transrenal ureteral occlusion with tissue adhesive and steel coil on the left side; contralateral defunctionalization of the kidney by transcatheter embolization of the renal artery. Indication: large vesicovaginal fistulae secondary to irradiation of vaginal cancer (75-year-old patient)

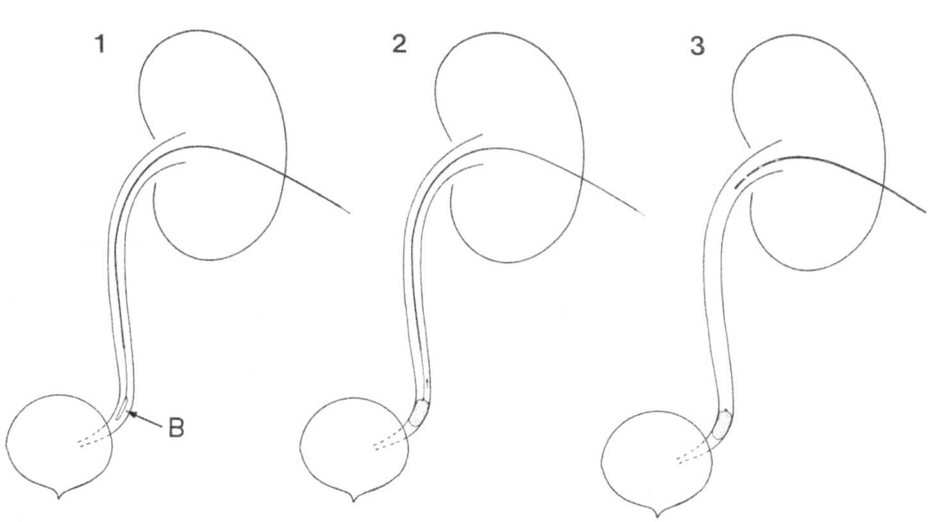

Fig. 11. Scheme for transrenal ureteral embolization using a detachable balloon filled with silicone

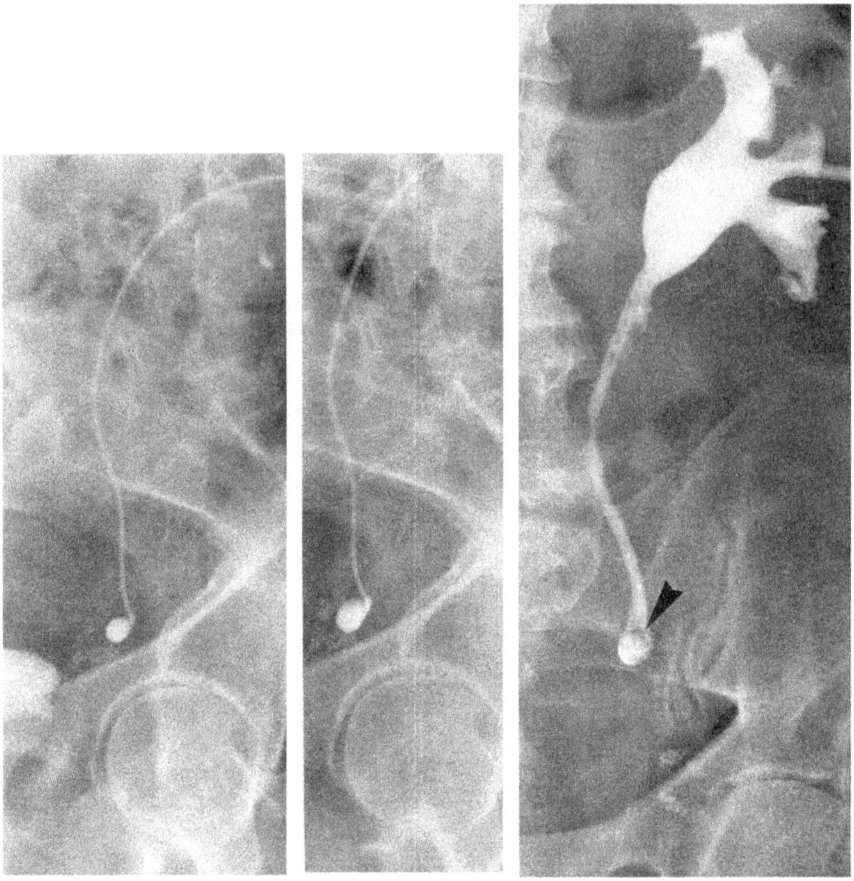

a b, c

Fig. 12a–c. Transrenal ureteral embolization with a detachable balloon. Indication: dysuria (painful pollakisuria) in advanced prostate cancer (right kidney defunctionalized by transcatheter embolization). **a, b** Balloon insertion and filling with silicone; **c** nephrostogram following detachment of the balloon

form of treatment even in patients with poor life expectancy. Under these circumstances permanent ureteral occlusion combined with PNS provides a reasonable alternative. The procedure can be performed bilaterally. If bilateral nephrostomy, however, is not tolerated or cannot be adequately attended, the contralateral kidney can be defunctionalized by transarterial embolization (*Günther* et al. 1979). A prerequisite for effective interruption of urinary flow is a well-functioning external nephrostomy drainage.

6.3 Results

6.3.1 Ureteral Embolization with Tissue Adhesive (Tables 11–13)

In 25 patients 28 transrenal ureteral embolizations (TUE) were performed:

Unilateral TUE	14 patients
Bilateral TUE	3 patients
Unilateral TUE combined with transcatheter embolization of the contralateral kidney	6 patients
Unilateral TUE combined with transcatheter embolization of the bladder	2 patients

All patients were inoperable either due to primary tumour extent, recurrent tumours or previous operations and irradiations for malignant tumors in the pelvis (Table 11). In 14 patients the contralateral kidney was non-functioning, while in two patients it had been surgically removed. Ten patients presented with large urinary fistulae (vesicovaginal 7, vesicorectovaginal 1, vesicosacrocutaneous 1, ureterovaginal fistulae 1). Fourteen patients had severe dysuria and four haematuria. One 75-year-old woman had total urinary incontinence (contracted bladder following irradiation). Of ten urinary fistulae, four ceased and six improved. Severe dysuria (painful pollakisuria, tenesmes) subsided in 11 of 12 instances. Haematuria could not be influenced satisfactorily by ureteral blockage (Table 12).

The effect of ureteral embolization with the tissue adhesive was insufficient in one case from the beginning. Long-term clinical follow-up studies as well as experimental results have shown that the tissue adhesive softens in the urine and can be expelled by ureteral peristalsis, especially if drainage is ineffective (*Günther* et al. 1980). In five of ten patients the ureter was reliably occluded after a follow-up period of 6–22 months. In the other patients the embolisate was partly or totally expelled (Table 13).

6.3.2 Ureteral Occlusion with a Detachable Balloon

This method was employed in three patients one of whom had painful dysuria due to inoperable prostate cancer (Fig. 12). The contralateral kidney was defunctionalized by transcatheter embolization. A second patient with bladder cancer presented with postoperative urinary fistula following ureterosigmoidostomy and a third with iatrogenic damage of the ureter secondary to deep anterior resection of the rectum resulting in abdominal urinoma and septicaemia.

In the first two patients, balloon occlusion of the ureter combined with PNS was the definitive treatment with perfect results. Dysuria and urinary fistulae stopped. In the third, the balloon ruptured during inflation but a second balloon effectively occluded the ureter and septicaemia subsided.

6.4 Complications

No severe complications were observed. Rupture of the small balloon was without sequelae and was due to the initial quality of the latex material used.

Table 11. Transrenal ureteral embolization (TUE): indications and underlying disease in 25 patients

I. Urinary fistulae (n = 10)	
Urethral cancer	1
Rectal cancer	1
Cervical cancer, following operation and irradiation	3
Cervical cancer, local recurrency	3
Inoperable cervical cancer	1
Vaginal cancer	1
II. Dysuria (tenesmes, painful pollakisuria, haematuria) (n = 14)	
Bladder cancer	11
Prostate cancer	1
Cervical cancer	1
Ovarial cancer and cystitis due to cystostatics	1
III. Total urinary incontinence (n = 1)	
Cervical cancer, radiogenic contracted bladder (pat. 75 years old)	1

Table 12. Effect of ureteral embolization on clinical symptoms

Symptoms	Cessation of complaints	Improved	Unchanged	No. of symptoms	No. of patients
Severe dysuria	7	4	1	12	15
Haematuria	–	1	7	8	
Incontinence	3	1	–	4	
Urinary fistulae	4	6	–	10	10

Table 13. Late results following transrenal ureteral embolization with tissue adhesive

Follow-up period (months)	No. of patients	Ureter occluded	Ureter partly patent	Ureter free	Embolisate expelled	
					Partly	Completely
6	2	–	2	–	2	–
7	1	1	–	–	1	–
9	1	1	–	–	1	–
10	1	1	–	–	1	–
11	2	1	–	1	1	1[a]
12	1	1	–	–	1	–
14	1	–	1	–	1	–
22	1	–	1	–	1	–
Total	10	5	4	1	9	1

[a] Tissue adhesive plus Gianturco coil

References

Alken P, Hutschenreiter G, Günther R, Marberger M (1981) Percutaneous stone manipulation. J Urol 125:463–466

Barbaric ZL, Wood BP (1977) Emergency percutaneous nephropyelostomy: Experience with 34 patients and review of the literature. AJR 128:453–458

Bigongiari LR, Lee KR, Moffat RE, Mebust WK, Foret J, Weigel J (1977) Percutaneous ureteral stent placement for stricture management and internal urinary drainage. AJR 133:865–868

Burnett LL, Roy JC Jr, Busch WH Jr (1976) A new method for percutaneous nephrostomy. Radiology 120:557–561

Debrun G, Lacour R, Caron JP, Hurth M, Comoy J, Keravel Y (1978) Inflatable and released balloon technique experimentation in dog – application in man. J Neurosurg 9:267–271

Fallon B, Olney L, Culp DA (1980) Nephrostomy in cancer patients: To do or not to do? Br J Urol 52:237–242

Fernström I, Andersson L (1977) Percutaneous puncture nephrostomy. In: Encyclopedia of Urology V/1, Diagnostic Radiology, pp. 129–174. Springer, Berlin-Heidelberg-New York 1977

Fernström I, Johansson B (1976) Percutaneous pyelolithotomy. A new extraction technique. Scand J Urol Nephrol 10:257–259

Finney RP (1978) Experience with a new double-J ureteral catheter stent. J Urol 120:678

Goldin AR (1977) Percutaneous ureteral splinting. Urology 10:165–168

Gonzalez-Serva L, Weinerth JL, Glenn JF (1977) Minimal mortality of renal surgery. Urology 9:253–255

Goodwin WE, Casey WC, Woolf W (1955) Percutaneous trocar (needle) nephrostomy in hydronephrosis. JAMA 157:891–894

Günther R, Altwein JE, Georgi M (1977) Feinnadelpunktion zur antegraden Pyelographie und perkutanen Nephropyelostomie. RöFo 127:439–441

Günther R, Schubert U, Bohl J, Georgi M, Marberger M (1978) Transcatheter embolization of the kidney with butyl-2-cyanoacrylate: experimental and clinical results. Cardiovasc Radiol 1:101–108

Günther R, Alken P, Altwein JE (1979) Perkutane Nephropyelostomie – Anwendungsmöglichkeiten und Ergebnisse. Fortschr. Röntgenstr. 128:720–726

Günther R, Alken P, Altwein JE (1979) Percutaneous nephropyelostomy using a fine needle puncture set. Radiology 132:228–230

Günther R, Alken P (1979) Perkutane Nephropyelostomie bei Kindern. Fortschr. Röntgenstr 130:586–589

Günther R, Altwein JE (1979) Perkutane Extraktion eines abgerissenen Nephrostomiekatheters. Fortschr Röntgenstr 130:121–122

Günther R, Alken P (1980) Interne Harnableitung durch antegrade Uretersplintung. RöFo 133:479–484

Günther R, Klose K, Bohl J, Marberger M (1980) Transrenale Ureterembolisation. Experimentelle und klinische Ergebnisse. RöFo 133:471–476

Günther R (1981) Perkutane Harnleiterembolisation. Technik, therapeutische Anwendung und Weiterentwicklung. Akt Urol 12:89–95

Haaga JR, Zelch MG, Alfidi RJ, Stewart BH, Daugherty JD (1977) CT-guided antegrade pyelography and percutaneous nephrostomy. AJR 126:621–624

Holden S, McPhee M, Grabstald H (1979) The rationale of urinary diversion in cancer patients. J Urol 121:19–21

Hutschenreiter G, Alken T, Klippel LF (1979) Ultraschallgesteuerte perkutane Nephrostomie. Urologe [A] 18:157–163

Karamcheti A, O'Donnel WF (1977) Percutaneous nephrolithotomy – innovative technique. J Urol 118:671–673

Kearney GP, Mahoney EM, Brown HP (1979) Useful technique for long-term urinary drainage by inlying ureteral stent. Urology 14:126–134

Lang EK (1981) Diagnosis and management of ureteral fistulas by percutaneous nephrostomy and antegrade stent catheter. Radiology 138:311–317

Levy JM, Potter WM, Stegman CJ (1979) A new catheter system for permanent percutaneous nephrostomy. J Urol 122:442–443
Link D, Leff RG, Hildell J, Drago JR (1979) The use of percutaneous nephrostomy in 42 patients. J Urol 122:9–10
Maar, K, Boeminghaus F, Blaschke R, Rick W (1977) In vitro Urinperfusion von Endoprothesen. Eine Studie zur Inkrustationstendenz in Kunststoffschläuchen. Urologe [A] 16:302–307
Mazer MJ, LeVeen RF, Call JE, Wolf G, Baltaxe HA (1979) Permanent percutaneous antegrade ureteral stent placement without transurethral assistance. Urology 14:413–419
Mulvaney WP (1960) The clinical use of Renacidin in urinary calcifications. J Urol 84:206–212
Murphy JT (1972): The history of urology. CC Thomas, Springfield, p 289
Pfister RC, Newhouse JH (1979) Interventional percutaneous pyeloureteral techniques. II. Percutaneous nephrostomy and other procedures. Radiol Clin N Am 17:351–363
Rupel E, Brown R (1941) Nephroscopy with removal of stone following nephrostomy for obstructive calculous anuria. J Urol 45:177–182
Sharer W, Grayhack JT, Graham J (1978) Palliative urinary diversion for malignant ureteral obstruction. J Urol 120:162–164
Smith AD, Reinke DB, Miller RP, Lange PH (1979) Percutaneous nephrostomy in the management of ureteral and renal calculi. Radiology 133:49–54
Smith AD, Lange PH, Miller RP, Reinke DB (1979b) Controlled ureteral meatotomy. J Urol 121:587–589
Spataro RF, Linke CA, Barbaric ZL (1979) The use of percutaneous nephrostomy and urinary alkalinization in the dissolution of obstructing uric acid stones. Radiology 129:629–632
Stables DP, Ginsberg NJ, Johanson ML (1978) Percutaneous nephrostomy series and review of the literature. AJR 130:75–82
Suby HI, Albright F (1943) Dissolution of phosphatic urinary calculi by the retrograde introduction of a citrate solution containing magnesium. N Engl J Med 223:81–91
Weiss EQ, Levya A, Hernandez A (1976) Treatment of lithiasis by forced injection of liquid and ureteral catheterization by the translumbar route. Int Surg 61:419–422
Weißbach L, Lunow R, Gebhardt M, Bastian HP (1979) Rasterelektronenmikroskopische Untersuchungen verschiedener Natur- und Kunststoffe nach Urineinwirkung in vitro. Urologe [A] 18:175–179
Zimskind PD, Fetter TR, Wilkerson JL (1967) Clinical use of long-term indwelling silicone rubber ureteral splints inserted cystoscopically. J Urol 97:840–844

Transhepatic Portal Catheterization with Pancreatic Venous Sampling Versus Angiography in the Localization of Pancreatic Functioning Tumors

R. Passariello[1], G. P. Feltrin[2], D. Miotto[2], S. Pedrazzoli[2], P. Rossi[1], and G. Simonetti[1]

Selective arteriography is a well-defined procedure in localizing functioning tumors of the pancreas; however, its diagnostic accuracy is rarely greater than 80% (*Clouse* et al. 1977; *Fugjii* et al. 1964; *Korobkin* et al. 1971; *Madsen* and *Hansen* 1970; *Robins* et al. 1973; *Stefanini* et al. 1974). To improve diagnostic accuracy in this field, transhepatic portal catheterization (TPC) has been introduced over the last few years (*Göthlin* et al. 1974; *Ingemansson* et al. 1975; *Lunderquist* and *Tylen* 1975; *Reichardt* and *Ingemansson* 1980) as a method of obtaining blood samples from pancreatic and peripancreatic veins for radioimmunologic assay of pancreatic hormone concentration.

Preliminary results using this technique to localize pancreatic functioning tumors have been reported previously (*Passariello* et al. 1978; *Pedrazzoli* et al. 1980). With this technique tumor localization is achieved by the demonstration of differences in hormone concentration in the pancreatic and peripancreatic veins. For this reason knowledge of the anatomy of pancreatic veins is fundamental for both the performance of sampling and the interpretation of results.

1 Anatomy of Pancreatic Veins

Pancreatic veins, as well as arteries, have a relatively complex anatomy (Fig. 1). Selective venography documents branches and anastomoses which are not so easily seen in anatomic preparations. There are two main venous systems: one in the

1 Department of Radiology, University of Rome, I-00161 Rome
2 Department of Radiology, University of Padua, I-35100 Padua

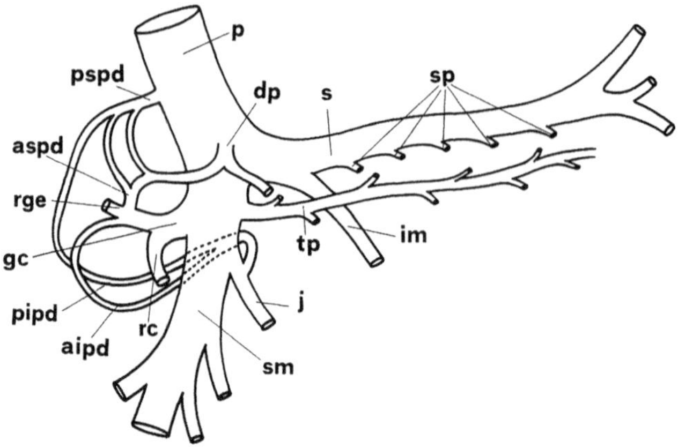

Fig. 1. Anatomy of the main pancreatic veins. *p,* portal vein; *pspd,* posterior superior pancreaticoduodenal vein; *aspd,* anterior superior pancreaticoduodenal vein; *aipd,* anterior inferior pancreaticoduodenal vein; *pipd,* posterior inferior pancreaticoduodenal vein; *rge,* right gastroepiploic vein; *gc,* gastrocolic trunk; *rc,* right colic vein; *sm,* superior mesenteric vein; *j,* first jejunal branch; *tp,* transverse pancreatic vein; *dp,* dorsal pancreatic vein; *s,* splenic vein; *im,* inferior mesenteric vein; *sp,* short pancreatic veins

head of the pancreas, the other in the body and tail of the pancreas. Anatomic variations are relatively rare at the level of the main venous trunks, while they are frequent in the more distal veins (*Douglas* et al. 1950; *Falconer* and *Griffiths* 1950; *Petrén* 1929; *Reichardt* and *Cameron* 1980). In the head of the pancreas the veins usually form an anterior and a posterior arcade, the former represented by the anastomosis of the anterior superior pancreaticoduodenal vein (ASPD) with the anterior inferior pancreaticoduodenal vein (AIPD) (Fig. 2).

The ASPD is a relatively constant vein which drains the most anterior portion of the head of the pancreas. It derives from the confluence of numerous small superficial branches crossing the pancreas from the periphery toward the center. It drains into the right gastroepiploic vein just prior to its confluence with the right colic vein to form the gastrocolic trunk (GC).

The GC enters the superior mesenteric vein (SMV) laterally below the head of the pancreas at a level 2–3 cm from the confluence of the SMV and the portal vein. The ASPD has anastomotic branches with AIPD and with the posterior superior pancreaticoduodenal vein (PSPD), as seen in venograms, and may also have connections with the dorsal pancreatic vein (DP) when this is present. The posterior arcade is made up by the anastomosis of the PSPD with the posterior inferior pancreaticoduodenal vein (PIPD).

The PSPD is the most frequent and the largest vein of the pancreatic venous system. It drains the posterior superior portion of the head of the pancreas and usually enters the portal trunk posteriorly above the head of the pancreas. Sometimes the PSPD is formed by two or more different trunks which enter the portal vein separately at a variable distance from the confluence between the latter vein and the SMV or directly at the confluence; the PSPD anastomoses not only with the PIPD but also with the ASPD and the DP.

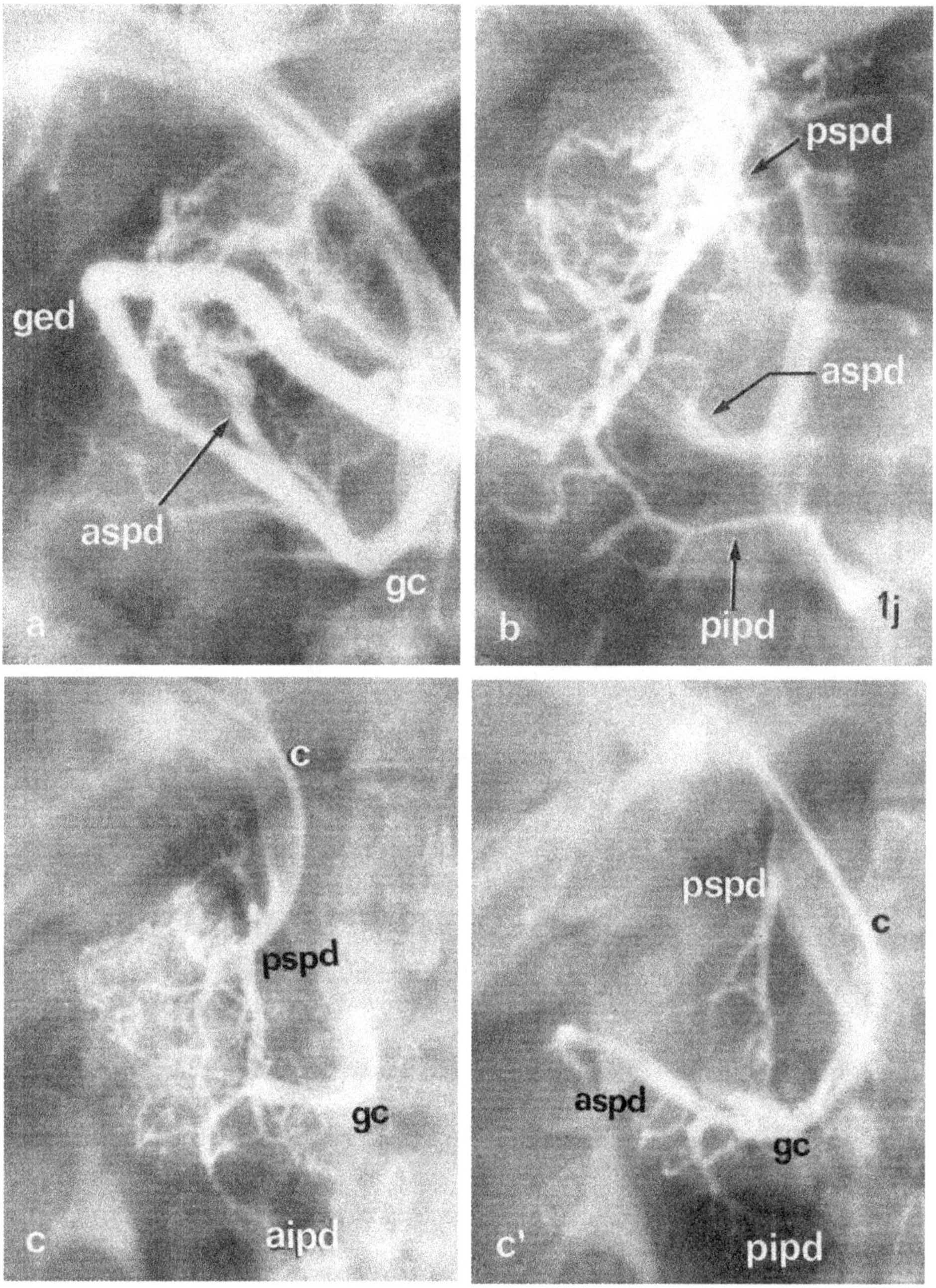

Fig. 2a–c′. In vivo anatomy of the veins at the level of the head of the pancreas. **a** Selective catheterization of the gastrocolic trunk (*gc*) with demonstration of the anterior superior pancreaticoduodenal vein (*aspd*) and of the right gastroepiploic vein (*ged*). **b** Selective venogram of the posterior superior pancreaticoduodenal vein (*pspd*) demonstrating anastomoses with the anterior superior pancreaticoduodenal vein (*aspd*) and with the posterior inferior one (*pipd*) which drains into the first jejunal branch (*1j*). **c, c′** Selective venograms of **c** the posterior superior pancreaticoduodenal vein and **c′** gastrocolic trunk. Communication between the veins of the head of the pancreas is evident. *c,* catheter; *pspd,* posterior superior pancreaticoduodenal vein; *aspd,* anterior superior pancreaticoduodenal vein; *gc,* gastrocolic trunk; *aipd,* anterior inferior pancreaticoduodenal vein

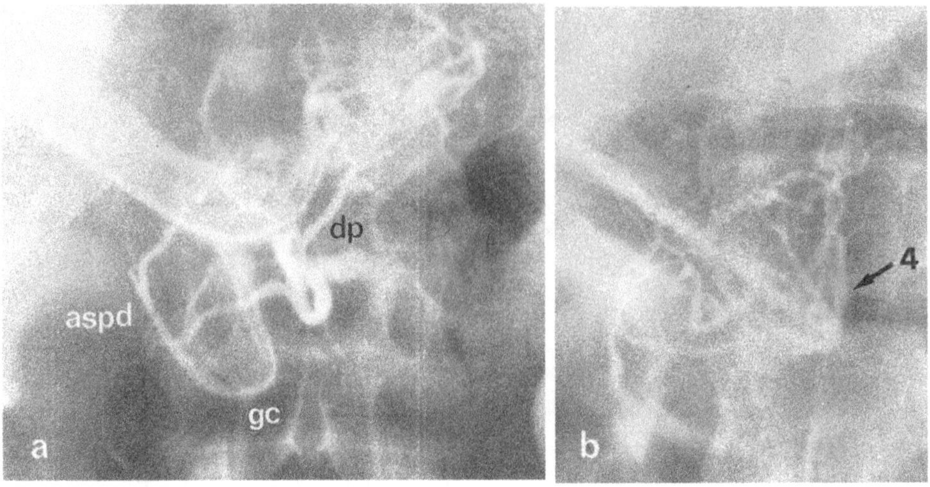

The AIPD is a relatively frequent and large vessel which drains the anterior, inferior portion of the head of the pancreas and part of the duodenum. The vessel passes posterior to the SMV and enters laterally into the first jejunal branch near its confluence with the SMV, or may form a common trunk with the PIPD.

The PIPD, which is not always present, is a small vessel which drains the inferior posterior portion of the head of the pancreas. As mentioned earlier, it forms a common trunk with the AIPD and enters into the first jejunal branch, but it may also flow directly into the SMV. Anastomoses are also present with the PSPD and the AIPD.

A less frequent vein of the head of the pancreas is the anterior pancreatico-duodenal vein, which derives from the anterior portion of the head of the pancreas and enters directly into the SMV. The DP is seldom encountered between the body and head of the pancreas (Fig. 3). This vein enters into the anterior inferior wall of the splenic vein at the junction with the SMV. Some right branches of the DP anastomose with the ASPD and PSPD, while the left branches anastomose with the transverse pancreatic vein (TP) and some of the short pancreatic veins (SP). The venous drainage of the body and tail of the pancreas is formed by the SP, draining to the splenic vein, and by the TP (Fig. 4), which runs along the inferior margin of the pancreas and ends in the splenic vein, or more often, in the lateral aspect of the SMV.

2 Materials and Methods

Between February 1976 and December 1980, 55 Patients were investigated in the Radiological Departments of the Universities of Rome and Padua by means of angiography and transhepatic portal catheterization (TPC) for possible pancreatic functioning tumors.

◄ **Fig. 3a, b.** In vivo anatomy of the veins of the pancreatic isthmus. **a** Selective venography of a short pancreatic vein arising from the splenic vein with evidence of multiple anastomoses with the dorsal pancreatic vein (*dp*), the anterior superior pancreaticoduodenal vein (*aspd*), and the gastrocolic trunk (*gc*). **b** Selective injection into an accessory pancreatic vein (*4*) connected with the venous system of the isthmus and head of the pancreas

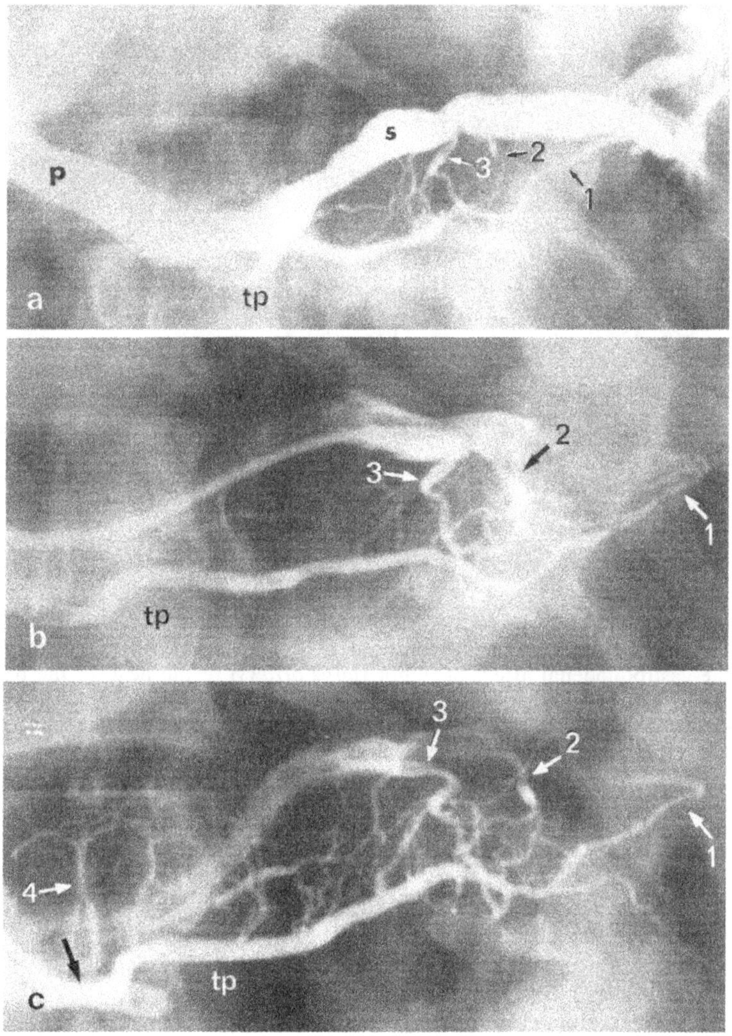

Fig. 4a–c. In vivo anatomy of the veins of body and tail of the pancreas. **a** Venography of the splenic vein (*s*) shows retrograde filling of multiple short pancreatic veins (1, 2, 3) connected with the transverse pancreatic vein (*tp*), *p*, portal vein. **b** The anastomoses between the veins of the body and tail of the pancreas are better demonstrated with selective venography of a short pancreatic vein (2) connected with other short veins (1, 3) and with the transverse pancreatic vein (*tp*). **c** Demonstration of the same anastomosis with selective injection into the transverse pancreatic vein (*tp*). Tip of catheter (*arrow*)

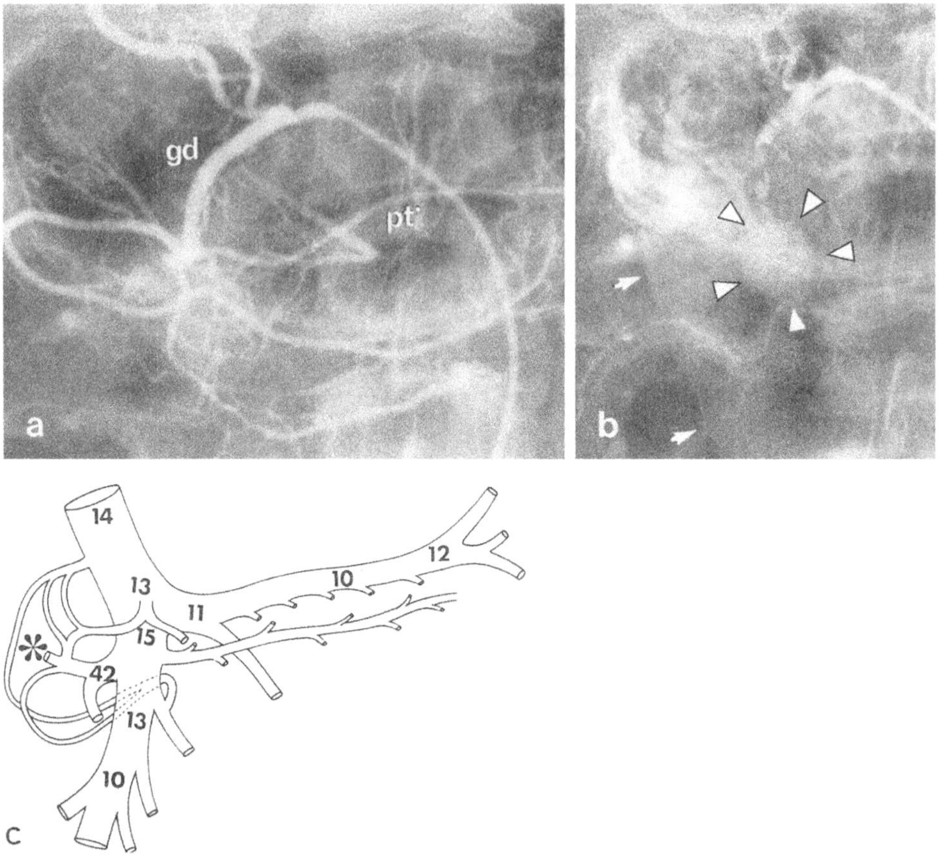

Fig. 5a–c. Insulin-producing tumor. **a, b** Demonstration with superselective arteriography of the gastroduodenal artery of tumor (*large arrows*) in the head of the pancreas. *Long arrows* point to the contour of the second duodenal tract. *pt′* = transverse pancreatic artery. **c** TPC confirms the presence of the tumor (*) in the head of the pancreas because of the high hormonal concentration (μU/ml) in the *gc* compared with the assays of other veins

Twenty-six patients had clinical symptoms suggesting hyperinsulinism (10 males and 16 females with ages ranging from 21 to 68 years, with an average age of 37.6 years). Twenty-eight had the Zollinger-Ellison syndrome (ZES) (23 males and 5 females with ages ranging 22–60 years, average age: 44.8 years). One patient had a suspected glucagonoma (22-year-old male).

In all the cases angiography preceded TPC, which was performed at the same time or a few days after angiography. In five additional patients TPC failed. In two of the cases it was impossible to catheterize the portal venous system while in the other three cases TPC was interrupted, once for technical reasons (occlusion of the catheter), and twice for clinical reasons (cardiovascular collapse in one case and hypoglycemic coma in the other).

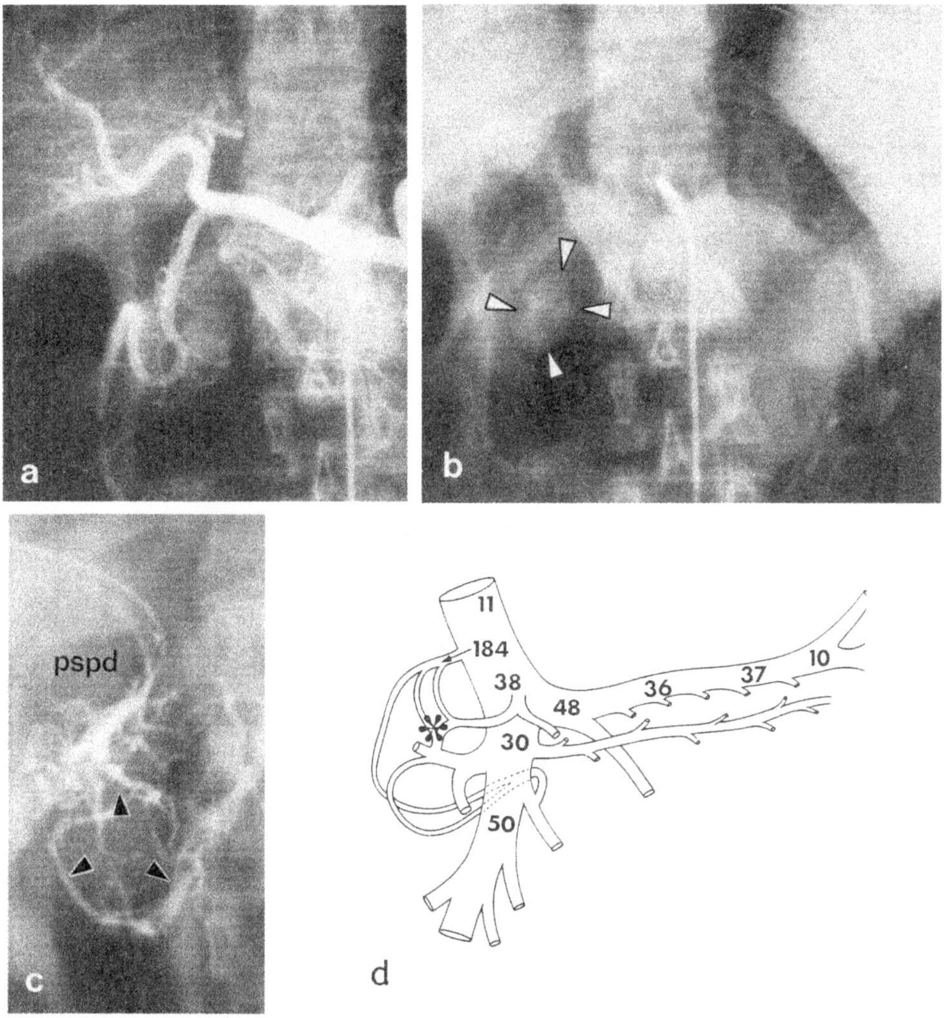

Fig. 6 a–d. Insulin-producing tumor. **a, b** Evidence of the tumor in the head of the pancreas at the selective arteriography of celiac trunk (*arrows*). **c** During TPC, the tumor is also evident with selective venography of the *pspd* revealing an avascular area (*arrows*). **d** The hormone assay confirms the presence of the tumor (*) in the head of the pancreas by the high hormonal concentration (μU/ml) in the *pspd*

In another six patients angiography revealed pancreatic endocrine tumors (five insulin- and one gastrin-producing tumor). These patients did not, however, undergo TPC because of the reliability of the angiographic pattern.

We had no lethal complications. One patient had hemoperitoneum which required emergency surgery 6 h after TPC. Almost all patients experienced pain in the right upper quadrant during the 12–24 h following TPC.

In 22 of 55 patients, pancreatic arteriography was performed with a superselective technique, while in the remaining 33 only celiac and superior mesenteric arteries were studied.

The technique of TPC was the following: After general sedation and local anesthesia, while the patient was in apnea, a polyethylene sheet needle (27 cm long, having an outer diameter of 1.14 mm) was inserted just anterior to the right midaxillary line, generally at a level corresponding to the 12th dorsal vertebra. Care was taken not to cross the lateral costophrenic angle.

The needle was horizontally directed toward the right portal branch, previously localized by the venous phase of arteriography, and was advanced to about 2–3 cm from the right paravertebral line. The metallic stylet of the needle was then withdrawn and the cannula was connected with a syringe containing contrast medium. The cannula was then slowly extracted, maintaining the syringe in aspiration. When a free flow of blood was obtained, a small test injection identified the cannulated vessel. If the tip of the cannula was seen in a major portal branch, a J-shaped guide wire was introduced deep into the portal system. The needle cannula was then exchanged for a 50 cm long catheter having one side hole close to its tip to facilitate the blood sampling.

To facilitate the manipulation and the eventual exchange of catheter and to reduce the friction between the catheter and the liver parenchyma, we used a polytetrafluoroethylene (Teflon) sheet over the catheter, extending from the skin to the portal trunk. At the beginning of the procedure 10–12 blood samples were drawn from the splenic, superior mesenteric, and portal veins. Then as many selective samples as possible were taken from the SP veins, GC, PSPD, first jejunal branch (J), TP, and DP. The number of samples depended on the anatomy, the technical success, the duration of the procedure, and the patient's cooperation and general condition. Selective catheterization of the pancreatic veins was usually obtained with the aid of curved guide wires.

In 6 of the 55 patients studied only nonselective samples were obtained. In the remaining 49 patients one or more selective samples from pancreatic veins were taken. With decreasing frequency, selective samples were obtained in the GC (43 cases), PSPD (28), SP (17), AIPD and PIPD (15), TP (8), DP (8), and ASPD (4); eight more samples were obtained in other cephalic pancreatic veins not well defined from an anatomic point of view.

A total of 131 selective samples were taken in the 49 patients, averaging 2.7 samples per patient.

Supplemental samples after pharmacologic stimulation of the pancreatic endocrine function were obtained in only a few cases. In two cases of suspected insulinomas the stimulation was performed with arginine (infusion of 0.5 g/min for 5 min and beginning of sampling 15 min after the end of the infusion), while in three cases of suspected Zollinger-Ellison syndrome (ZES), secretin was used in two cases and bombesine in one case (infusion of 5 units/kg secretin or 10 mg/kg per minute for 5 min of bombesine and beginning of sampling 20 min after the end of the infusion). At the end of the procedure, a fibrin sponge plug was introduced through the catheter into the liver to prevent bleeding from the puncture site. The methods for radioimmunologic assay of pancreatic hormones have been previously reported (*Pedrazzoli* et al. 1980).

3 Results

3.1 Insulin-Producing Tumors and β-Cell Hyperplasia (Figs. 5 and 6)

Of 26 patients 21 showed insulin-producing tumors when operated on, while two patients had β-cell hyperplasia. In 19 cases a single insulinoma was found and in two cases two tumors were found in the same pancreatic region. The tumors were localized in the head of the pancreas in ten patients, in the body of the pancreas in four patients, between the body and tail of the pancreas in three, and in the tail of the pancreas in four patients. The tumor diameter ranged from 4 mm to 35 mm (average: 12.2 mm). β-cell hyperplasia was present in the head of the pancreas in one patient and in the other one in the entire pancreas.

The remaining three patients could not be appraised for the following reasons:

One patient died due to diabetes mellitus 3 months after TPC and the autopsy did not reveal functioning tumors in the pancreas.
One patient was operated on but no lesion was found.
One patient refused surgery.

In the verified cases, angiography and TPC demonstrated different levels of accuracy (*Galen* 1975), presented in Tables 1 and 2.

The diagnostic results of selective and nonselective samples were as follows:

Selective pancreatic samples suggested tumor localization in 10 of 12 patients (83%), and nonselective in 16 of 23 (69%).
Selective samples localized the lesion in four cases where the nonselective were negative; the opposite was obtained in only one case.
The localization of tumors or β-cell hyperplasia was achieved with only selective samples in four cases, with only nonselective samples in ten cases, and on the basis of both sets of data in six cases.

Table 1. Accuracy of angiography and TPC

		True positive	True negative	False positive	False negative
Insulinomas and β-cell hyperplasia (n = 23)	Angiography	9	0 [a]	1 [b]	13 (+1)
	TPC	20	0 [a]	3 [b]	(2)
Gastrinomas, metastases, micronodular hyperplasia (n = 24)	Angiography	9	6	2 [b]	7 (+1)
	TPC	15	5	3 [b]	1 (+1)

[a] The absence of true negative diagnoses depends on the high reliability of clinical patient selection in this field.
[b] The number includes cases of concomitant false negative diagnoses, reported in parentheses in the false negative column.

Table 2. Accuracy of statistical data [a]

		Sensi-tivity	Speci-ficity	Diagnostic accuracy	Predictive value of positive tests	Predictive value of negative tests
Insulinomas, and β-cell hyperplasia	Angiography	39	[b]	39	90	[b]
(n = 23)	TPC	91	[b]	87	87	[b]
Gastrinomas, metastases, micronodular	Angiography	53	75	68	82	43
hyperplasias (n = 24)	TPC	88	63	83	83	71

[a] Approximation of percentage values
[b] Values not estimable due to the absence of true negative diagnoses in the series

Stimulation with arginine was useful in one case, while in the other it caused a false positive diagnosis. The other diagnostic errors were obtained once with selective and once with nonselective samples.

Altogether there were three diagnostic errors:

One patient with an insulinoma in the tail of the pancreas had a high hormonal concentration in the SMV. Presumably the tumor was drained by the TP vein which, however, was not selectively catheterized.

One patient previously operated upon with tail resection had β-cell hyperplasia in the remaining pancreas but false tumor localization to the body.

One patient with a tumor in the head of the pancreas had it falsely localized to the tail. No selective samples were obtained from veins draining the head in this patient.

3.2 Zollinger-Ellison Syndrome (ZES) (Fig. 7)

Of the 28 patients studied, 24 were verified at surgery or autopsy. In four cases medical treatment alone was given on the basis of the diagnostic results.

In the 24 verified patients the following conditions were revealed:

1. Gastrinomas – 13 cases
   six single tumors in the pancreas (five in the head and one in the body)
   two multiple tumors in the pancreas, three and two tumors, respectively, in the pancreatic head
   three single tumors in the duodenal wall (two in the second and one in the third portion)
   two tumors in one patient in the second portion of the duodenum
   one single tumor in the first jejunal loop.

The tumors had a diameter ranging from 8 to 42 mm (average 16.5 mm).

2. one case of micronodular hyperplasia in the entire pancreas
3. two cases of single lymph node metastases present at the level of the pancreatic head, without evidence of primary tumors
4. two cases of hepatic metastases (one single in the right lobe and one multiple in both lobes) without evidence of primary tumors
5. six cases of a normal pancreas with or without retained antrum syndrome submitted to total gastrectomy with or without partial or total pancreatectomy.

In these 24 patients angiography and TPC revealed different accuracy levels, reported in Tables 1 and 2. TPC with sampling of blood gave the following results:

Selective samples correctly localized the lesions in 14 of 16 patients (87%), while nonselective samples gave accurate information in only 15 of the 24 patients (62%)

Selective samples localized the lesions in five cases where the nonselective were negative. The opposite was never observed

The localization of tumors and metastases was obtained with only selective samples in five cases, with only nonselective samples in six cases and on the basis of both in nine cases

The samples taken after stimulation with secretin and bombesine gave an indication of the site of the lesion in two cases and failed in one. However, in both cases where stimulation gave the correct indication, the data obtained were not diagnostic.

In four cases of diagnostic errors two were obtained with selective and two with nonselective samples and consisted of:

Two false localizations of a tumor in the head of the pancreas; one patient was found to have a normal pancreas at surgery and one at autopsy

One false localization of a tumor to the tail of the pancreas in a patient where operation showed gastrinoma of the head of the pancreas

One failure to localize a gastrin-producing tumor in the first jejunal loop

3.3 Glucagon-Producing Tumor (Fig. 8)

The only glucagon-producing tumor in the series was malignant and had a diameter of 40 mm. Both angiography and TPC localized the tumor correctly.

Statistical Analysis of TPC Diagnostic Results

Plasma concentration values of pancreatic hormones assayed in selective and nonselective samples were evaluated from a statistical point of view in order to ascertain:

1. Significance of the obtained results
2. Different significance of selective and nonselective samples
3. Minimum significance threshold of values with respect to localization

The following hormone concentration values were tabulated thus in all verified cases:

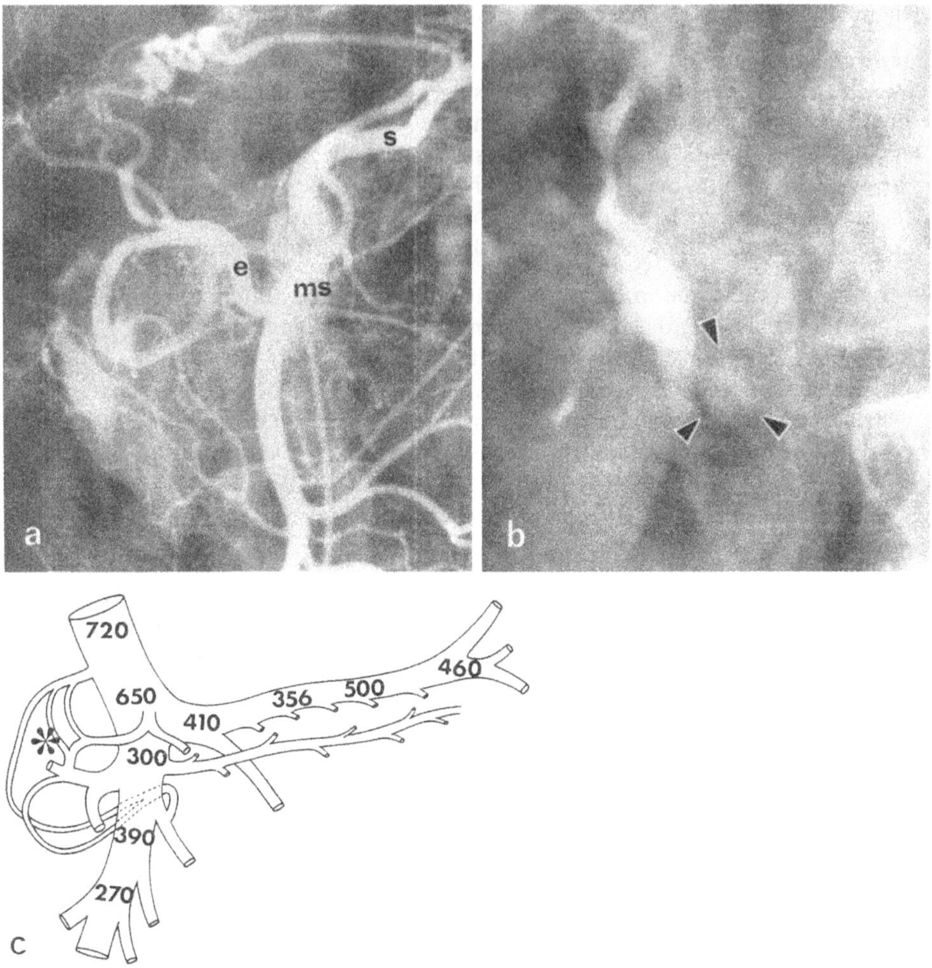

Fig. 7a–c. Gastrin-producing tumor. **a** Selective arteriography of the superior mesenteric artery (*ms*) shows the anomalous origin of the hepatic (*e*) and splenic (*s*) arteries. **b** In the capillary phase a hypervascularized area, less than 1 cm in diameter is present in the head of the pancreas (*arrows*). **c** Venous sampling confirms the presence of the functioning tumor (*) at the level of the head of the pancreas by the demonstration of peak values of hormone concentration (pg/ml) in the portal vein

Value A: hormonal concentration in the pancreatic vein draining the tumor (when this vein had been selectively catheterized)

Value B: peak of hormonal concentration in the main peripancreatic vein contiguous to the pancreatic region containing the tumor

Value C: average value of hormonal concentration in the samples obtained in a main peripancreatic vein distant from the tumor

Value D: hormonal concentration obtained in the sample taken more distally in the SMV, peripheral to the entrance of the first jejunal branch; this was considered the basal value.

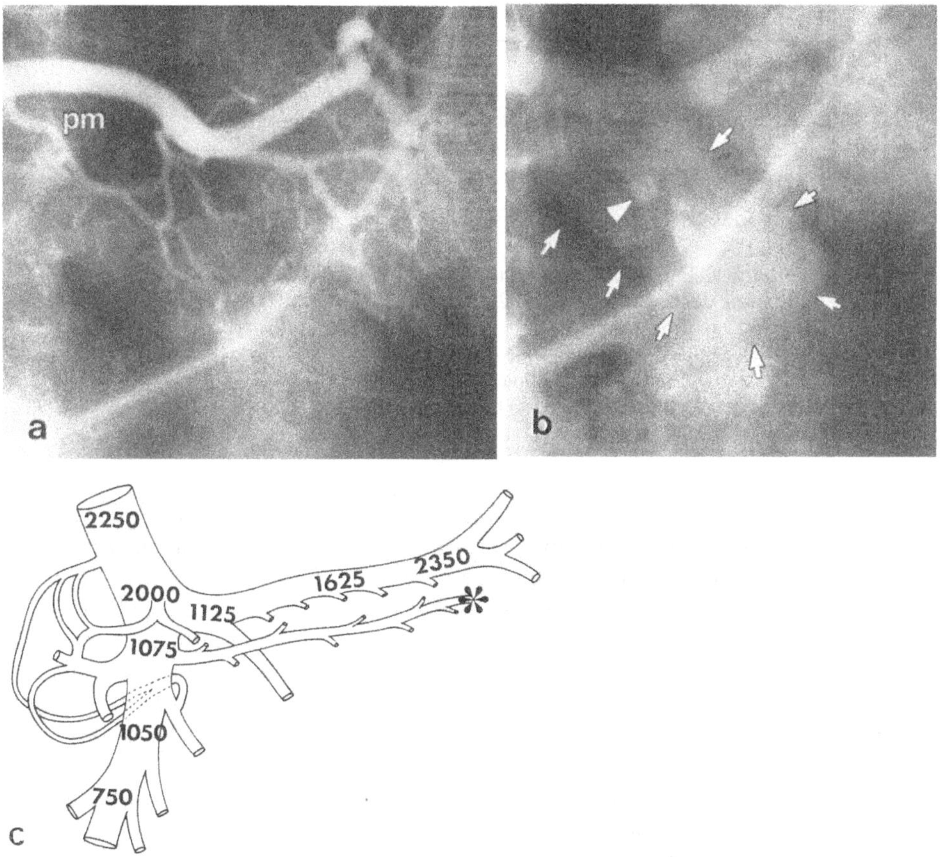

Fig. 8a–c. Glucagon-producing tumor. The tumor is strongly suspected at selective splenic arteriography. **a** In the arterial phase wide pancreatic arteries are observed (*pm*, pancreatica magna artery). **b** In the capillary and venous phases a homogenous pathologic blush appears at the level of the tail (*arrows*) **c** Blood samples confirm the presence of a high glucagon concentration (pg/ml) in the distal splenic vein

For the statistical evaluation, the values A, B, and C were expressed as a percentage of the D value.

The following tests of statistical significance were performed on the obtained data:

Test 1: comparison between values A and D
Test 2: comparison between values B and D
Test 3: comparison between values C and D
Test 4: comparison between values A and B
Test 5: comparison between values A and C
Test 6: comparison between values B and C
Test 7: research to find the significant threshold values of the investigation, i.e., to define the minimum relative hormonal concentration values necessary to confirm that a functioning tumor could be present in a certain pancreatic region.

Table 3. Significance tests of hormonal concentration values

Tests	Insulin-producing tumors		Gastrin-producing tumors	
	Differences (%)	Significance	Differences (%)	Significance
1	610.0±294.3 [a]	$P<0.0001$	563.6±486.2	$P<0.02$
2	268±127.6 [b]	$P<0.0005$	202.1±112.5	$P<0.05$
3	181.9±199	n.s. [c]	129.6± 68.1	n.s. [c]
4	267.0±129	$P<0.01$	272.0±234.7	$P<0.05$
5	Due to the lack of significance of test 3, both these tests are significant			
6	to the same degree as tests 1 and 2			
7	226.2± 50.6	$P<0.01$	171.3± 42.8	$P<0.02$

[a] Only the cases having values < 1000% have been considered.
[b] Only the cases having values < 600% have been considered.
[c] No significance

The various tests were considered with regard to insulinomas and gastrinomas and the results are reported in Table 3. Special consideration was taken with test 7, i.e., the definition of the significant threshold value.

Differences of up to 180% relating to basal values were considered to be without significance in *insulin-producing* tumors (Table 3, test 3), while differences of 270% were significant for tumor presence. Peak values in the main vein contiguous to the tumor ranging from 150% to 300% were therefore evaluated. A statistically significant difference ($P<0.01$) was found to have a value of 226.2% of the basal value (Table 3, test 7).

The peak value observed in the main peripancreatic vein contiguous to the *gastrin-producing* tumor was also evaluated, since the value in the vein draining the tumor was usually very high and the values in the main vein distant from the tumor were usually low and not significant. The evaluation was made between the value of 120% (not significant) and 270% (significant) (Table 3, tests 3 and 4). A statistically significant difference ($P<0.02$) was found at 171.3% of the basal value (Table 3, test 7).

4 Discussion and Conclusions

Transhepatic portal catheterization (TPC) with venous blood sampling from pancreatic and peripancreatic veins is a diagnostic method which is quite easy to perform. In our series we observed 8% with technical failure and less than 1% with major complications. Our data are similar to those obtained by *Burchardt* who mentioned 4% with technical failure and 2% with complications.

In our experience, TPC has a diagnostic accuracy greater than angiography: our results were 87% and 39%, respectively, for insulin-producing tumors and β-cell hyperplasia, and 83% and 63% for ZES (Figs. 9, 10).

Transhepatic portal catheterization also permitted us to suspect or ascertain islet cell hyperplasia, which cannot be detected by angiography.

Arteriography was more accurate when performed with superselective techniques than when performed with celiac and superior mesenteric angiography.

The low diagnostic accuracy of angiography in our series, if compared with that reported in the literature (*Clouse* et al. 1977; *Fugjii* et al. 1974; *Korobkin* et al. 1971; *Robins* et al. 1973; *Stefanini* et al. 1974) results mainly from two factors:

Most of the patients included in our series represent a select group of cases unsuccessfully studied in other hospitals

With the high diagnostic accuracy of TPC we found no reason to repeat angiography with superselective techniques, but instead carried out the more diagnostic TPC.

It is true that arteriography gave a high number of false negative reports in this series, but there were few false positive diagnoses and therefore there was a high predictive value for a positive test. Furthermore, in one case of insulinoma arteriography modified a TPC localization error. For these reasons and because of the useful information on vascular anatomy, angiography always has to be performed before TPC in cases of suspected functioning tumors of the pancreas.

Transhepatic portal catheterization is imperative when angiography is doubtful or negative, but may not be performed in patients where an insulinoma or glucagonoma is clearly defined at angiography.

On the other hand, TPC has to be performed in patients with ZES, even in the presence of a positive angiogram. The reason for this is the frequent occurrence of multifocal lesions or of diffuse hyperplasia of the islet cells in this syndrome.

From a practical and statistical point of view, the more selective the samples, the more accurate are the TPC results; in fact, in compiling insulin- and gastrin-producing tumors and hyperplasias, selective samples disclosed the site of the lesion in 85% of the cases non selective in 65.5%. Statistical evaluation of hormonal concentration values showed in relation to basal values more significant values in tumor-draining veins than the peak values in the main peripancreatic veins contiguous to the tumor.

Analysis of the results obtained (Table 3) permits us to conclude that a high statistical probability exists of localizing an insulin- or gastrin-producing tumor in a particular pancreatic region when:

1. The hormonal concentration in a pancreatic vein is 5.7–6.1 times higher than the basal value
2. There is peak value of hormonal concentration in a main peripancreatic vein contiguous to this region which is 2.1–2.7 times higher than the basal value
3. There is a hormonal concentration in the pancreatic vein draining the tumor 2.7–2.8 times higher than the peak value obtained in the main peripancreatic vein

In spite of the remarkable differences in the absolute values in hormonal concentration between insulin- and gastrin-producing tumors it is evident that the percentage values are similar. The same similarity is also evident when the significant threshold values necessary to localize a functioning tumor are defined. For insulinomas and gastrinomas these were 2.3 and 1.8 times higher, respectively, than the basal values. Thus, the presence of a peak of hormonal concentration in a main

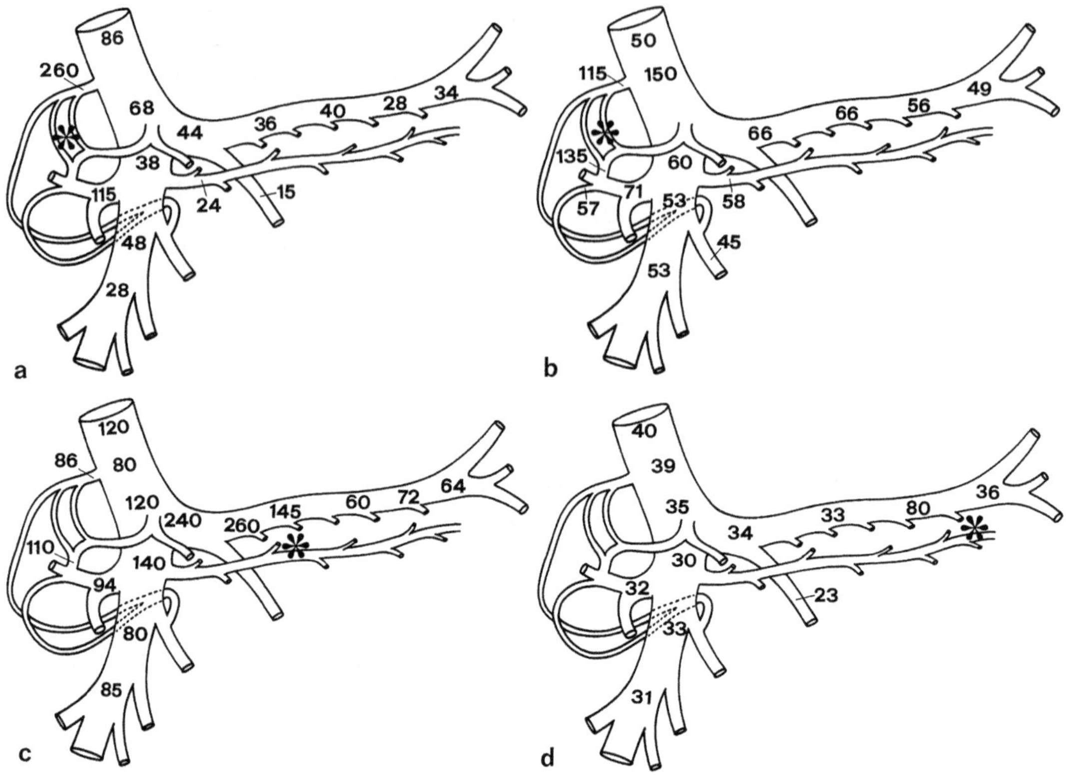

Fig. 9a–d. Four cases of insulin-producing tumors not evident at angiography and localized by TPC (hormonal values are rexpressed in μU/ml). **a** Tumor in the head of the pancreas; high values of insulin concentration in the *pspd, gc,* and vena portae. **b** Tumor in the head of the pancreas; high values of insulin concentration in the *pspd, aspd,* and vena portae. **c** Tumor in the body of the pancreas; peak values of insulin concentration in the proximal tract of the splenic vein. **d** Tumor in the tail of the pancreas; peak value of insulin concentration in the distal part of the splenic vein

peripancreatic vein 2.3 and 1.8 times higher, respectively, than the basal value represents the minimum value to confirm (with a margin of error of 1% and 2%, respectively) that an insulin- or a gastrin-producing tumor drains into the vein in question.

These data give us a significant possibility of localizing a pancreatic functioning tumor even when during TPC the tumor-draining vein had not been selectively catheterized.

It is important to consider that the many anastomosing channels between the pancreatic veins can give different concentration values of the hormones when the tip of the catheter is at slightly different levels. We observed this phenomenon in two cases of insulin-producing tumor. In the first, localized to the tail of the pancreas, the TP was the predominant draining vein of the tumor, while in the splenic vein hormonal concentration values were almost normal.

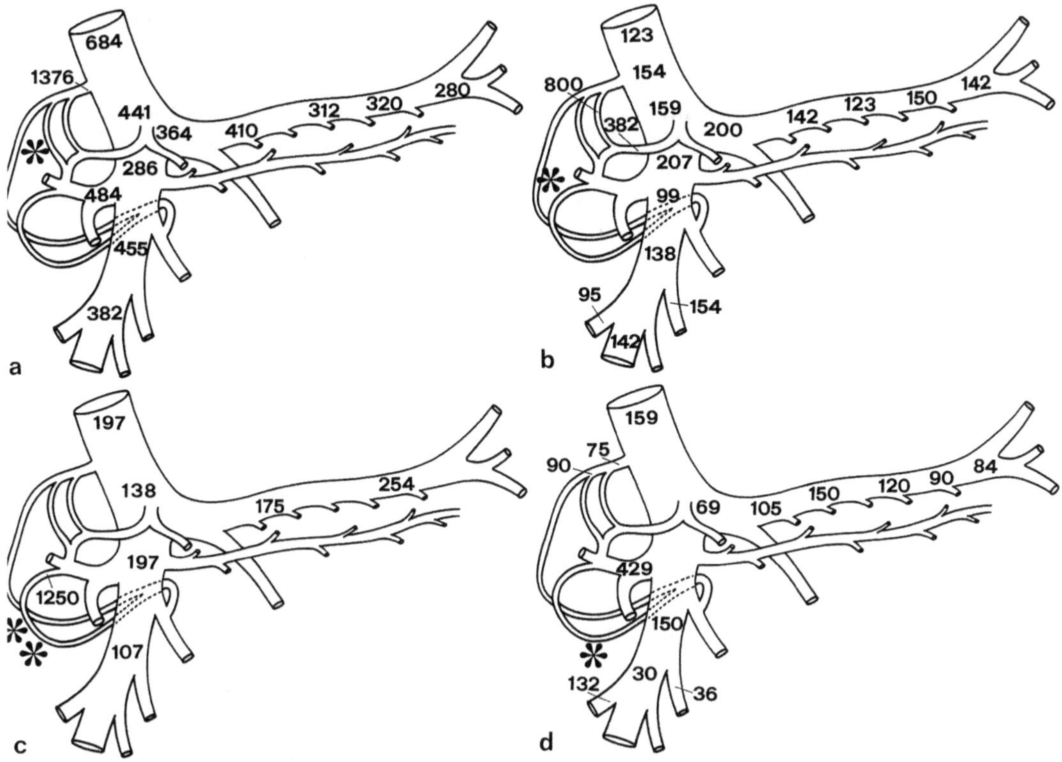

Fig. 10 a–d. Four cases of gastrin-producing tumors not evident at angiography and localized by TPC (hormonal values are expressed in pg/ml). **a** Tumor in the head of the pancreas; high values of gastrin concentration in the *pspd* and vena portae. **b** Tumor in the second part of the duodenum; high values of gastrin concentration in the *aspd.* **c** Double tumor in the second part of the duodenum; high values of gastrin concentration in the *aipd.* **d** Single lymph node metastasis at the level of the head of the pancreas (without surgical evidence of the primary tumor localization); high values of gastrin concentration in the *gc*

In the second patient the tumor localized in the head of the pancreas gave high hormonal concentration values in the GC while the value was almost normal in the PSPD.

In spite of the significance demonstrated for nonselective samples, selective samples should always be obtained and should also, when possible, be multiple from the same pancreatic region.

More complex and less positive is the evaluation of TPC in the presence of a β-cell hyperplasia or of diffuse micronodular gastrin-producing hyperplasia (or tumors).

In fact, while TPC revealed the case of β-cell hyperplasia present in the head of the pancreas, the procedure gave a false diagnosis in the case of diffuse hyperplasia. Moreover, high gastrin values were present in one patient with micronodular hyperplasia as well as in two patients with a normal pancreas, and in two patients with retained antrum syndrome. More data are necessary in this field and more patients will have to be studied and appraised to obtain results of statistical significance.

In spite of the limited number of cases studied, we have found that the venous samples after pharmacologic stimulation are not so useful that they justify a prolonged procedure. We find it more important to take a large number of selective pancreatic samples which influence diagnostic accuracy.

5 Summary

Fifty-five patients with suspected pancreatic functioning tumors were studied by angiography and transhepatic portal catheterization (TPC) with pancreatic venous sampling for radioimmunological hormone assay. Tumors producing insulin was present in 21, glucagon in 1, and gastrin in 17 patients. Functioning hyperplasia of the pancreas was present in 3 patients, while the remaining 13 were not verified or presented a normal pancreas. TPC revealed a diagnostic accuracy superior to angiography: 87% vs 39% in the insulin-producing tumors, and 83% vs 63% in the gastrin-producing tumors.

Analysis of the data obtained with TPC showed that the hormonal levels in tumors are statistically significant for their localization. The more selective the samples were in the pancreatic veins, the more accurate were the TPC results. On the other hand, the values obtained in islet cell hyperplasia were not significant. Ultimately the samples obtained after pharmacologic stimulation of the endocrine pancreas proved of little value.

Acknowledgement. We thank Roberto Pasquali-Lasagni, M.D. and Claudio Modini, M.D. for statistical analyses and Miss Patrizia Cesari for secretarial assistance.

References

Burchardt F (1979) Percutaneous transhepatic portography. I. Technique and application. AJR 132:177–182

Clouse ME, Costello P, Legg MA, Soeldner SS, Cady B (1977) Superselective angiography in localizing insulinomas of the pancreas. AJR 128:741–746

Douglass BE, Baggenstoss AH, Hollinshead WH (1950) The anatomy of the portal vein and its tributaries. Surg Gynecol Obstet 91:562–576

Falconer CWA, Griffiths E (1950): The anatomy of the blood vessels in the region of the pancreas. Br J Surg 37:334–344

Fugjii K, Yagata S, Saski R, Ohneda A, Shoji T, Suzuki J (1974) Arteriography in insulinomas. AJR 120:634–647

Galen RS (1975) Productive value of laboratory tests. Am J Cardiol 36:536–544

Göthlin J, Lunderquist A, Tylén U (1974) Selective phlebography of the pancreas. Acta Radiol [Diagn] (Stockh) 15:474–480

Ingemansson S, Lunderquist A, Lundquist I., Lovdahl R, Tibblin S (1975) Portal and pancreatic vein catheterization with radioimmunologic determination of insulin. Surg Gynecol Obstet 141:705–711

Korobkin MT, Palubinskas AJ, Glickman MG (1971) Pitfalls in arteriography of islet-cell tumors of the pancreas. Radiology 100:319–328

Lunderquist A, Tylén U (1975) Phlebography of the pancreatic veins. Radiology 15: 198–202

Madsen B, Hansen ES (1970) Correlation between angiographic diagnosis and of pancreatic insulinomas. Br J Radiol 43: 185–192

Passariello R, Rossi P, Simonetti G, Di Paolo A (1978) Catheterisme portal trans-hépatique pour la localization des tumeurs secrétantes du pancréas. Ann Radiol (Paris) 21: 485–490

Pedrazzoli S, Feltrin G, Oddi G, Miotto D, Pasquali C, Cevese PG (1980) Usefulness of transhepatic portal catheterization in the treatment of insulinomas. Br J Surg 67: 557–561

Petrén T (1929) Die Arterien und Venen des Duodenums und des Pancreaskopfes beim Menschen. Z Anat Entwickl.-Gesch. 90: 234–277

Reichardt W, Cameron R (1980) Anatomy of the pancreatic veins. A post mortem and clinical phlebographic investigation. Acta Radiol Diagn 21: 33–41

Reichardt W, Ingemansson S (1980) Selective vein catheterization for hormone assay in endocrine tumors of the pancreas. Techniques and results. Acta Radiol Diagn 21: 169–176

Robins JM, Bookstein JJ, Oberman HA, Fajans JJ (1973) Selective angiography in localizing islet cell tumor of the pancreas. Radiology 106: 525–528

Stefanini P, Carboni M, Patrassi N, Basoli A (1974): Beta-islet cell tumors of the pancreas. Results of a study on 1067 cases. Surgery 75: 597–609

New Topics in Embolization

Effects of Central, Peripheral, or Capillary Type of Occlusion in Animal Models Simulating Tumor Embolization

G. W. Kauffmann[1], G. Richter[1], J. Rassweiler[1], and R. Rohrbach[2]

1 Departments of Diagnostic Radiology, University of Freiburg, D-7800 Freiburg/i. Br.
2 Department of Pathology, University of Freiburg, D-7800 Freiburg/i. Br.

1 Introduction

Embolization is one of the new therapeutic methods in radiology. It has found acceptance for special indications such as emergency treatment of intractable bleeding (*Athanasoulis* 1980; *Kauffmann* et al. 1979; *Rösch* et al. 1972). However, tumor embolization is still controversial, since long-term results are so disappointing that few indications for palliative treatment are left. Even in a case with hematuria caused by renal cell carcinoma, recurrent hemorrhage is reported following Gianturco-Anderson-Wallace coil occlusion (*Flamm* et al. 1981). Failure of tumor embolization is caused by collaterals and recanalization of occluded arteries. Therefore only temporary reduction of tumor size is achieved: collaterals provide continuing growth in the periphery of the tumor. Clearly the possibilities of tumor embolization are not exhausted so long as the tumor periphery is not primarily occluded. Up to now there has been no medium that reaches the periphery but avoids venous propagation. All media especially developed for embolization, like the Gianturco-Anderson-Wallace coil, detachable balloons, etc., allow occlusion only of the main renal arteries. Ethibloc is the first substance especially developed for peripheral transport (besides occlusion of the pancreatic duct). Its special properties for reducing efficiency of collateral supply were examined and compared with the effect of Gelfoam powder, Butyl cyanoacrylate/Lipiodol and ligation of the renal artery.

2 Material and Methods

In a first step, the specific properties (viscosity, occlusion mechanism, radiodensity) of Gelfoam powder, Butyl 2-cyanoacrylate and Ethibloc were tested in vitro to optimize their transcatheteral application. In a second step, *normal rat kidneys* were embolized with increasing amounts of embolization volume to detect the influence on the extent of renal necrosis. The normal rat kidney is a model with very few collaterals. In a third step, *renal rat tumors* induced by dimethylnitrosamine (DMN) were used to examine the efficiency of capillary occlusion on tumor embolization. In particular the problems of preembolic estimation of the embolization quantity and the behavior of the various embolization media in the presence of a.v. shunts were studied. In a fourth step, capillary embolization was performed in *canine kidneys* with Ethibloc/glucose to simulate clinical angiographic techniques using balloon catheters.

2.1 Embolization Media

2.1.1 Gelfoam Powder[1]

Contents: Bovine collagen. Available as sterilized powder (1 g). Preferred embolization mixture: 1 g Gelfoam powder mixed with 30 ml Urografin 76% (Schering,

1 Upjohn, Heppenheim, FRG

Berlin). Occlusion mechanism: Mechanical blood stasis followed by intravascular thrombus formation. Gelfoam particles form the matrix for platelet aggregation (*Berenstein* and *Kricheff* 1979; *Greenfield,* 1980; *Jander* and *Russinovich* 1980; *Rassweiler* et al. 1980).

2.1.2 N-Butyl 2-Cyanoacrylate

Contents: N-Butyl 2-cyanoacrylate (NBC). Available in 0.5-ml vials (Histoacryl[2]) with methylene blue. Preferred embolization mixture: NBC is mixed with the iodized oil Lipiodol Ultra-fluid (Byk-Gulden, Konstanz) in equal amounts (1 : 1). Occlusion mechanism: Polymerization in contact with ionized substances (*Dotter* et al. 1975; *Günther* et al. 1978).

2.1.3 Ethibloc[3]

Contents:

The 7.5-ml vial contains an alcoholic solution (60%) of:
210 mg Zein (corn protein)/ml alcohol – occluding agent
162 mg Sodium amidotrizoate/ml alcohol – contrast medium
145 mg Oleum papaveris/ml alcohol – prevents file formation
6 mg Propylene glycol/ml alcohol – disinfectent

Available for clinical embolization in sterilized 7.5 ml syringes. Occlusion mechanism: Precipitation of the alcohol-soluble Zein in contact with blood (*Kauffmann* et al. a 1980; *Rassweiler* et al. 1980). Ethibloc was developed especially for embolization purposes (*Bücheler* et al. 1978) and admitted by the Bundes Gesundheits Amt Berlin for preoperative embolization of renal cell carcinoma (admission number: 342.000).

2.2 Laboratory Experiments

In laboratory experiments the following properties of the three embolization media were examined:

Radiodensity
Viscosity
Passage through angiographic catheters

Radiodensity was calculated by the iodine content of the embolization mixture and differences were visualized by radiographs taken of equal amounts of the embolization media (*Rassweiler* et al. 1980). *Viscosity* was determined by the Stokes viscosimeter at 20 ° and 37 °C. Various substances (contrast medium, normal saline, 40% glucose, 70% alcohol) were injected before and after the embolization material in order to test the *passage of the embolization media* through angiographic tubes. Different catheters with decreasing inner diameter (1.0–0.4 mm) were used.

---

2 Braun-Dexon, Melsungen, FRG
3 Ethicon, Hamburg, FRG

2.3 Normal Rat Kidney

In 400 male Wistar Rats (300–400 g) under pentobarbital anesthesia (48 mg Nembutal/kg body weight, i.p., Abbott, Bad Segeberg) the left carotid artery was surgically exposed and a 2 F thrombectomy catheter (Fogarty, Edwards Lab., Santa Ana, California) – after removal of the inner coil and the balloon tip – was introduced. Following laparotomy the catheter was manipulated into the left renal artery and fixed with a double ligation (silk 4/0) to avoid reflux. Rising embolization volumes from 0.01 ml to 0.07 ml of the three embolization agents were injected (Table 1). The control group had ligation of the main renal artery and 40% glucose perfusion (0.05 ml). Half of the animals were killed immediately, the other half 2 months later. Possible complications (reflux, pulmonary embolism) were studied by varying the injection conditions (e.g., overembolization, no ligation). Results of peripheral or capillary embolization were compared with central-type occlusion represented by ligation of the main renal artery. All treated kidneys were examined microscopically (hematoxylin-eosin, Goldner, Elastica van Gieson, Masson, PAS stains). All injections were performed with tuberculin syringes with a graduation of 0.01 ml and an accuracy of 0.01 ml ± 0.003.

Table 1. Review of animal experiments in capillary embolization. Different embolization media were tested in vasoocclusion of normal rat kidney, DMN-induced renal rat tumors, and canine kidney

Experimental group	Embolization volume	Gelfoam powder	NBC/ Lipiodol	Ethibloc	Control groups
Normal rats	0.01 ml	–	–	20	–
($n=400$)	0.02 ml	20	20	20	–
	0.03 ml	20	–	20	–
	0.04 ml	20	–	20	–
	0.05 ml	20	20	40	–
	0.06 ml	20	–	20	–
	0.07 ml	–	20	20	–
Ligation		–	–	–	10
Glucose	0.05 ml	–	–	–	10
Complications	Variable	10	20	30	–
Tumor rats					
($n=221$)					
smaller and medium-sized tumors (M)	0.05 ml to 0.15 ml	32	31	46	–
Ligation		–	–	–	14
Glucose		–	–	–	5
larger tumors (L)	0.15 ml to 0.5 ml	25	28	28	–
Ligation		–	–	–	12
Canine kidney ($n=15$)	4.5 ml to 6.0 ml	–	–	15	–

2.4 Renal Rat Tumors

In 500 female Wistar rats (90–120 g) renal tumors were induced by a single intraperitoneal injection of dimethylnitrosamine (60 mg DMN/kg body weight following 4 days of protein-free diet; *Magee* and *Barnes* 1962; *Murphy* et al. 1966). In the 221 surviving animals, bilateral renal tumors developed after an incubation period of 6–7 months. Selective catheterization of the renal artery was performed as previously described. Exact preembolic determination of the embolization volume by contrast medium perfusion could not be performed as the reduced excretory renal function leads to an extreme sensitivity to contrast medium injections. For rough estimation of the necessary embolization volume, the size of the surgically exposed tumor in comparison to normal rat kidney is taken. Tumors are classified and subdivided into two groups:

Tumors with a size smaller than the six fold normal rat volume (M = medium)
Tumors with a larger volume (L = large)

Half of the animals were killed immediately after embolization, the other half were used for follow-up study, with an average survival time of 65 days. In order to study the animals as long as possible, the larger of the bilateral renal tumors was embolized. The same embolization media were tested, and the control group again received ligation of the main renal artery and 40% glucose perfusion (Table 1). Microscopic sections of each tumor kidney were examined.

2.5 Dog Experiments

In 8 mongrel dogs (16–32 kg) under pentobarbital anesthesia (300 mg Nembutal/kg body weight, i.v.) both renal arteries were catheterized successively with a 5–7 F balloon catheter with Seldinger's technique. With the following embolization schedule, 15 canine kidneys were embolized with Ethibloc:

Preinjection of 40% glucose (20%–30% of estimated embolization volume)
Ethiblochinjection
Following injection of 40% glucose (3–4 ml)

The embolization volume needed was estimated by preembolic perfusion of the renal artery with contrast medium via the inflated balloon catheter: After injection of 4–6 ml contrast medium, parenchymal stain began, which was taken as indicating the necessary embolization volume (Table 1). After occlusion of the right kidney, embolization was performed on the left side 3–5 months later. This was followed by necropsy and microscopic examination of both kidneys and the lungs to exclude pulmonary embolism.

3 Results

3.1 Laboratory Experiments

3.1.1 Radiodensity

Radiodensity of Gelfoam powder is obtained by adding Urografin 76% (1 g/30 ml). This mixture corresponds to 340 mg iodine/ml. The mixture of NBC/Lipiodol (1 : 1) that we used corresponds to 240 mg iodine/ml. The sodium amidotrizoate in Ethibloc corresponds to 120 mg iodine/ml. A modified Ethibloc with a radiodensity increased to 210 mg iodine/ml is in preparation. This is achieved by exchanging iodized oil (i.e., Lipiodol Ultra-fluid) for the oleum papaveris (Fig. 1).

3.1.2 Viscosity

The viscosity of NBC/Lipiodol is remarkably low (14 cP at 20 °C). The viscosity of Gelfoam powder/Urografin 76% is ten times higher (100 cP at 20 °C); the measurements showed the inconstant rheological behavior of this particle suspension (*Rassweiler* et al. 1980). The viscosity of Ethibloc is high at 20 °C (760 cP). However, it decreases considerably at 37 ° (200 cP), which improves the injection properties (Fig. 2).

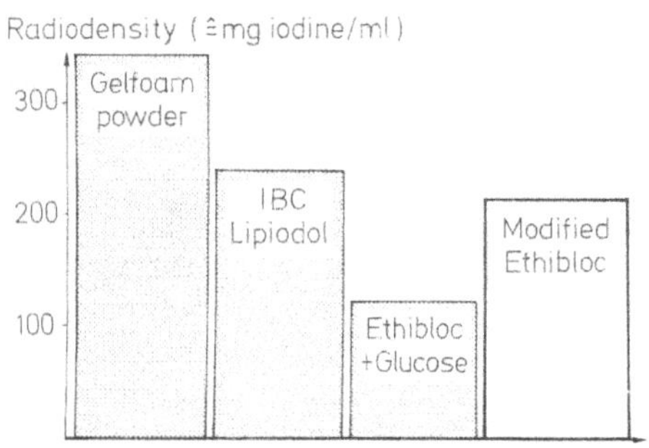

Fig. 1. Diagram of radiodensities of Gelfoam powder/Urografin 76%, NBC/Lipiodol, Ethibloc and contrast enhanced Ethibloc

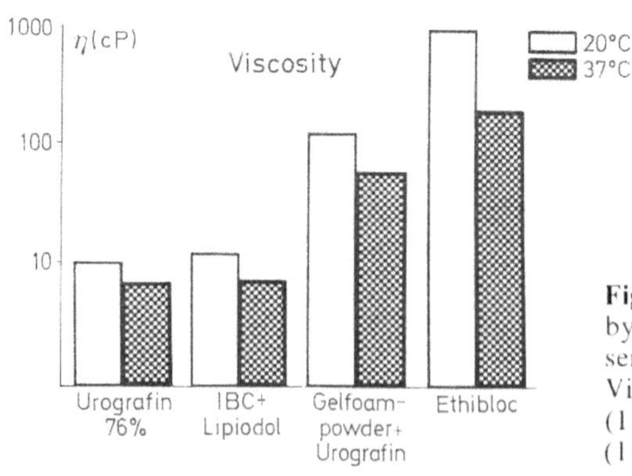

Fig. 2. Diagram of viscosity as determined by Stoke's viscosimeter documented on semi-logarithmic paper in centipoise (cps): Viscosity of Urografin 76%, NBC/Lipiodol (1 : 1), Gelfoam Powder/Urografin 76% (1 : 30), and Ethibloc at 20 ° and 37 °C

3.1.3 Passage Through Angiographic Catheters

According to different occlusion mechanisms, the various embolization media need pre- and postembolic injection with different substances to avoid catheter occlusion.

Gelfoam powder forms a thrombus only in contact with blood, therefore preinjection of special substances is not necessary. Clearing of the catheter with normal saline or contrast medium is quite possible.

Since the polymerization of *NBC* is catalyzed by anions, *pre*injection of 40% glucose is necessary to delay polymerization time and guarantee catheter passage. If NBC is mixed with Lipiodol (1 : 1), the mixture remains stable and polymerization time in contact with blood is prolonged by a factor of 10 (*Cromwell* and *Kerber* 1979; *Rassweiler* et al. 1980). If NBC is mixed with 40% glucose, the mixture does not remain stable and polymerization starts within 10 min (*Günther* et al. 1978; *Thelen* et al. 1976). Even traces of anions (i.e., in contrast medium, normal saline, blood, or hydroxylions in 40% glucose) definitely lead to polymerization of NBC and irreversible occlusion of the catheter. Therefore *post*injection must be performed first with small amounts of the unpolar Lipiodol, followed by 40% glucose. The Lipiodol prevents the contact of NBC/Lipiodol with the 40% glucose, and the following glucose injection prevents reflux of Lipiodol into the aorta.

*Pre*injection of normal saline or contrast medium leads to precipitation of *Ethibloc,* resulting in irreversible occlusion particularly of smaller catheters (2 F). In larger tubes, preinjection of 5%–10% glucose prevents early precipitation.

With the 2 F catheters we used, only preinjection of 40% glucose or 70% alcohol guarantees normal passage of Ethibloc through the catheter. These observations are more comprehensible if the *mechanism of Ethibloc precipitation* is explained: The main part of the occlusion gel is the non-water-soluble corn protein Zein in alcoholic solution (60%). Since the alcohol dissolves in watery media, Zein precipitates in contact with blood and forms a cast with the consistency of chewing gum. A 40% glucose solution is able to delay this precipitation because of its osmotic effect:

Table 2. Microscopic demonstration of the embolization medium using constant amounts of Ethibloc (0.05 ml) and increasing 40% glucose preinjection

Localization of Ethibloc	Quantity of preinjected glucose (40%)				
	0.01 ml	0.04 ml	0.08 ml	0.1 ml	0.12 ml
Segmental arteries	+ +	+ +	+ +	+ +	+ +
Glomerula	(+)	+ +	+ +	+ +	+ +
Venules	–	–	+	+ +	+ +
Renal vein	–	–	–	(+)	+ +
Pulmonary embolism	–	–	–	–	+ +

Microscopic demonstration of Ethibloc:
– no
(+) rarely
\+ 10%–50%
\+ + more than 50%

Glucose molecules aggregate water molecules, which then are not available for solution of the alcohol. Speed of precipitation corresponds to surrounding glucose concentration. This effect is used to guarantee controlled propagation of the Ethibloc within the arterial system down to the capillary bed. Table 2 shows the influence of increasing amounts of preinjected 40% glucose on the Ethbloc transport within the renal vascular system. If low amount of 40% glucose is pre-injected, only segmental arteries are reached. If too much 40% glucose is preinjected and the capillaries are filled with glucose, precipitation takes place within the venous system, and venous passage with pulmonary embolism occurs. *Post*injection of 40% glucose clears the catheter, but a residue of precipitated Ethibloc remains in the tube; 70% alcohol clears even those wall-adherent rests. Therefore each catheter should be rinsed with 70% alcohol before resterilization.

The volume of preinjected 40% glucose is dependent on the quantity of Ethibloc needed. The volume of postinjected 40% glucose is dependent on the volume of the catheter.

3.2 Animal Experiments

3.2.1 Normal Rat Kidney

In preliminary experiments the vascular volume of the rat kidney was determined as 0.12–0.14 ml (*Rassweiler* et al. 1980). As the arterial volume of the kidney is calculated as 20%–30% of the total vascular volume (*Boylan* et al. 1970), we use only embolization volumes rising from 0.01 ml up to 0.07 ml.

Gelfoam Powder. Gelfoam particles (10–100 μm) are not found within glomerular capillaries; only preglomerular arterioles were reached. It does not form a homogenous cast within all vessels, some arteries are only occluded partially (Fig. 3). Overembolization (more than 0.05 ml embolization volume) results in hilar paravasation. In the long-term group the well-known tendency for recanalization is seen (Fig. 4). However, it decreases with rising amounts of Gelfoam powder (0.05 or 0.06 ml).

Butyl 2-Cyanoacrylate. NBC/Lipiodol is seen in glomerular and rarely in peritubular venules. Over-embolization does not result in hilar paravasation, but in venous migration (Fig. 5). Two months later a 8–11 mm necrotic shrunk kidney is found. Since Lipiodol stays included within the polymerized NBC, postembolic shrinkage of the embolized kidney can be documented radiologically. On microscopic sections the embolized organs are completely necrotic, but contain multiple foreign-body granulomas surrounding the embolization medium.

Ethibloc. Following an embolization volume of 0.05 ml, the embolization medium is found homogenously distributed within the arterial system and the glomerular capillaries. Using higher volumes of Ethibloc, hilar paravasation occurs, comparable to that with Gelfoam powder. Two months after embolization, total necrosis of the kidney is found if 0.05 ml ("ideal volume") of Ethibloc has been used (Fig. 6). Completely necrotized hyaline glomerula are found surrounded by

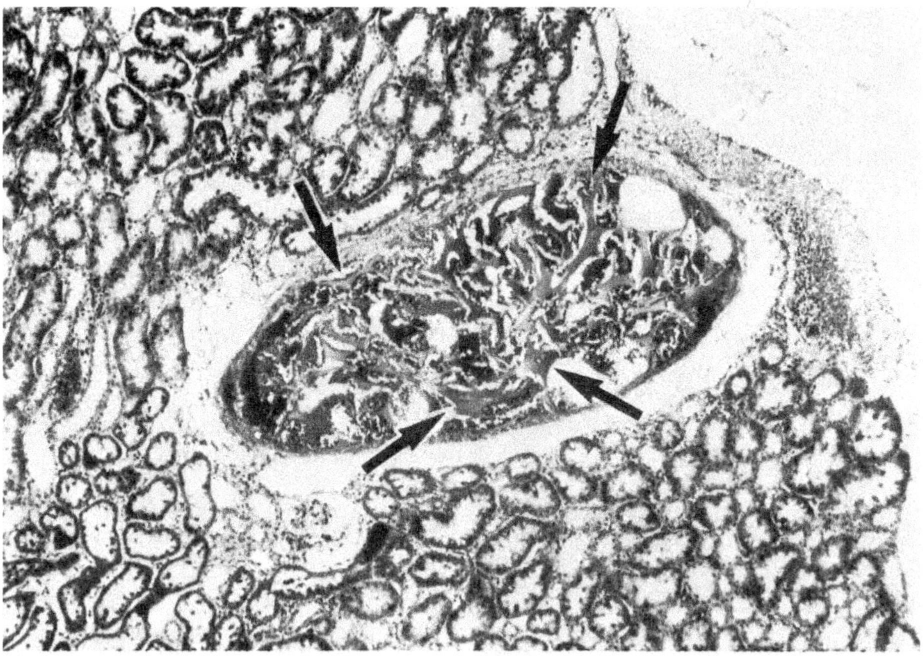

Fig. 3. Microscopic section of a segmental artery 1 day after embolization with partial filling of gelfoam: Bizarre formation of Gelfoam particles (*arrows*), aggregated thrombus, the remaining lumen (one third) is filled with red blood cells. HE×80

granulation tissue. Ethibloc can be identified down to segmental arteries, which are still completely occluded. No foreign-body reaction can be found (Fig. 6). If more than 0.06 ml of embolization medium is injected, unspecific round-cell inflammatory reaction occurs (Fig. 7).

Ligation. Two months after ligation, the kidney has shrunken to 12–15 mm, one third of the original size. Calcium deposits are seen throughout the organ, and cross sections and microscopic sections show scattered intact parenchymal areas, particularly in the renal cortex (Fig. 8).

With Gelfoam powder, NBC, and Ethibloc, effectivity is dependent on injected quantity. Best results are achieved with an embolization volume of 0.05–0.06 ml for all three embolization media (Fig. 9).

3.2.2 Dimethylnitrosamine-induced Renal Rat Tumors

3.2.2.1 Macro- and Microscopic Tumor Classification

Using the WHO classification (WHO 1976), we found interstitial mesenchymal tumors and adenocarcinomas with varying differentiation (*Hard* 1971 a, b, c). Accessory arterial vessels representing parasitic blood supply are documented macro- and microscopically (Fig. 10).

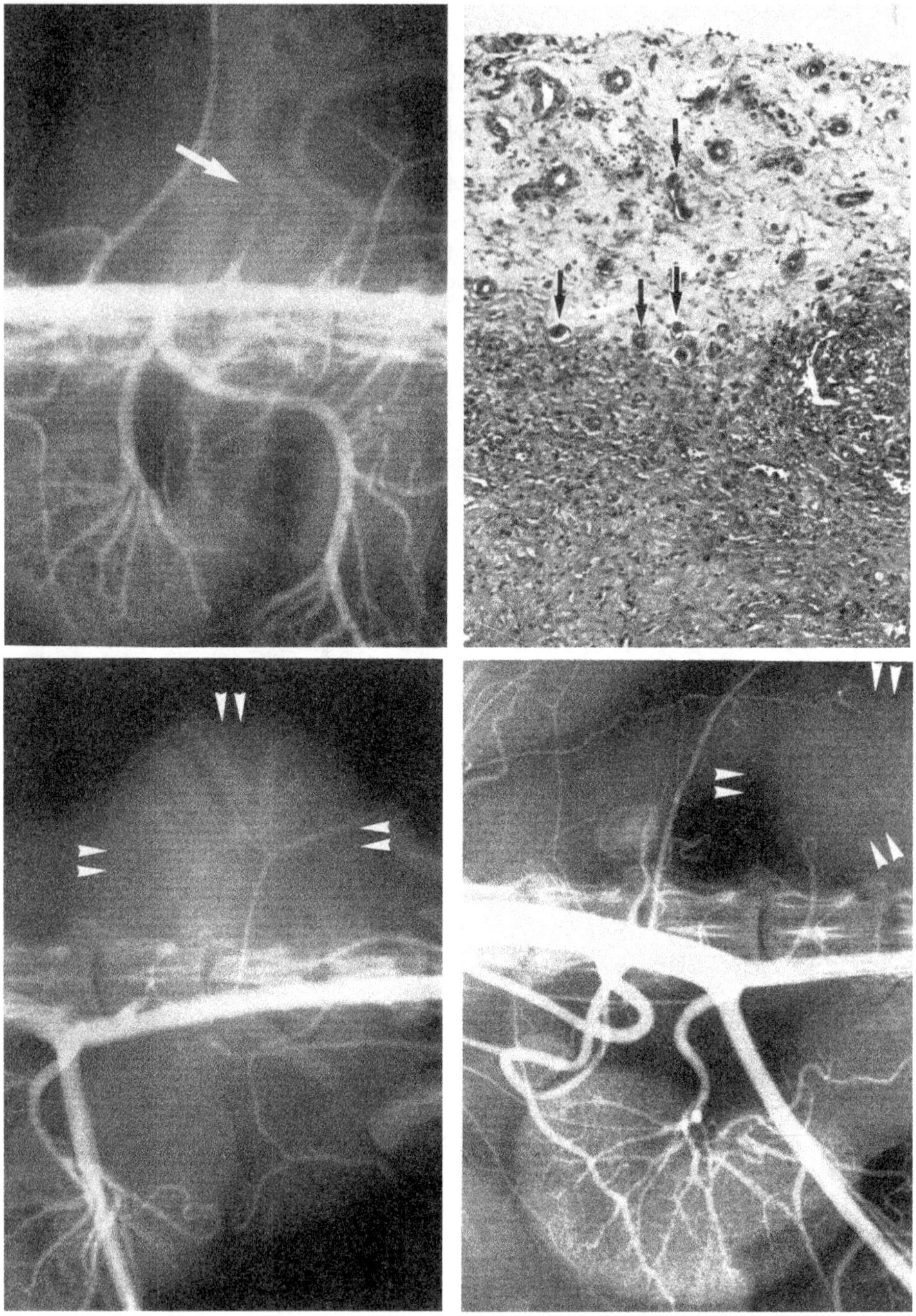

Fig. 4a–d. Tendency of recanalization of gelfoam. **a** Angiographic control 15 min after embolization: Proximal occlusion of the left renal artery, embolized kidney still faintly contrasted (*arrows*). **b** Control angiogram 7 days later: The left renal artery filled with contrast medium to the renal hilus without intrarenal vessels. **c** Same kidney 2 months later. Recanalization of intrarenal arteries as well as shrunken kidney (*arrows*). **d** Microscopic section of the same kidney: Necrosis of central parenchyma, cortex with still intact parenchyma, capillaries filled with red blood cells (*arrows*). HE × 25

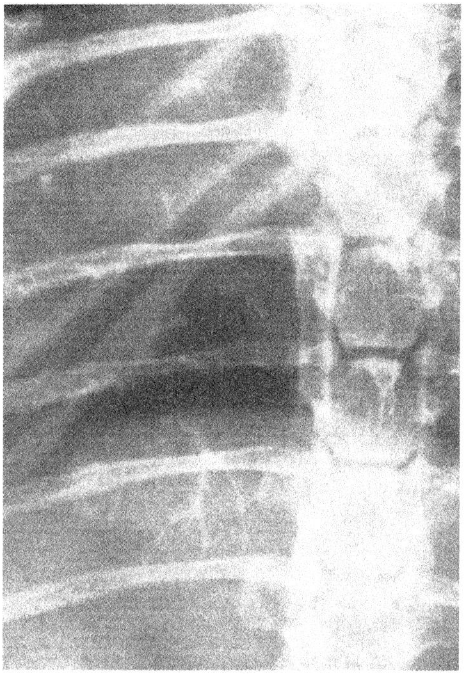

Fig. 5. Radiograph of the lung with NBC/ Lipiodol in the lung artery of the right lower lobe following embolization of the left kidney with 0.06 ml

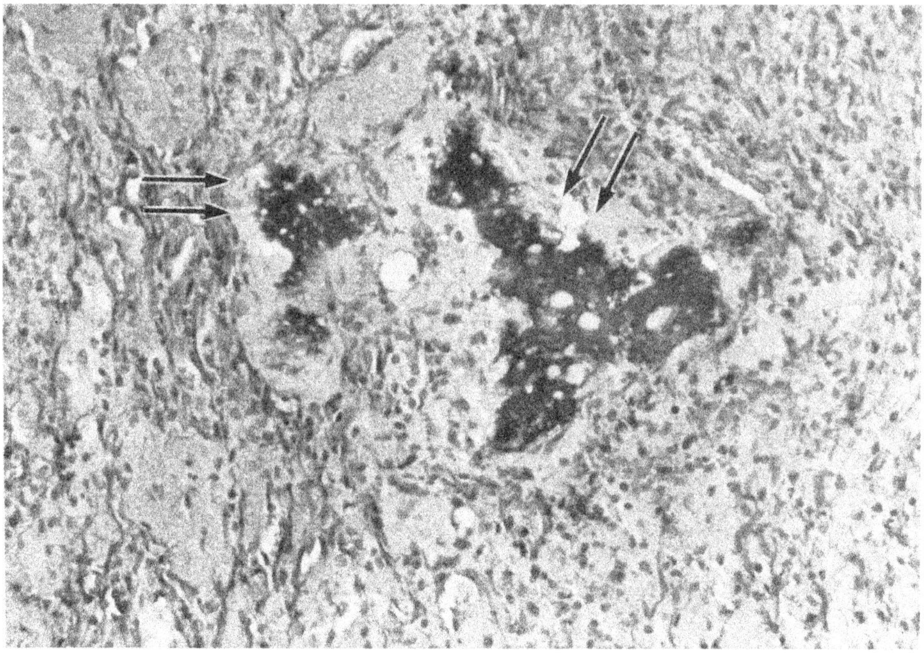

Fig. 6. Microscopic documentation of Ethibloc 2 months after embolization. Partial atrophy of the surrounding tissue. Residue of Ethibloc (*arrows*) within an arcuate artery organized by granulation tissue. No foreign-body reaction. EVG × 160

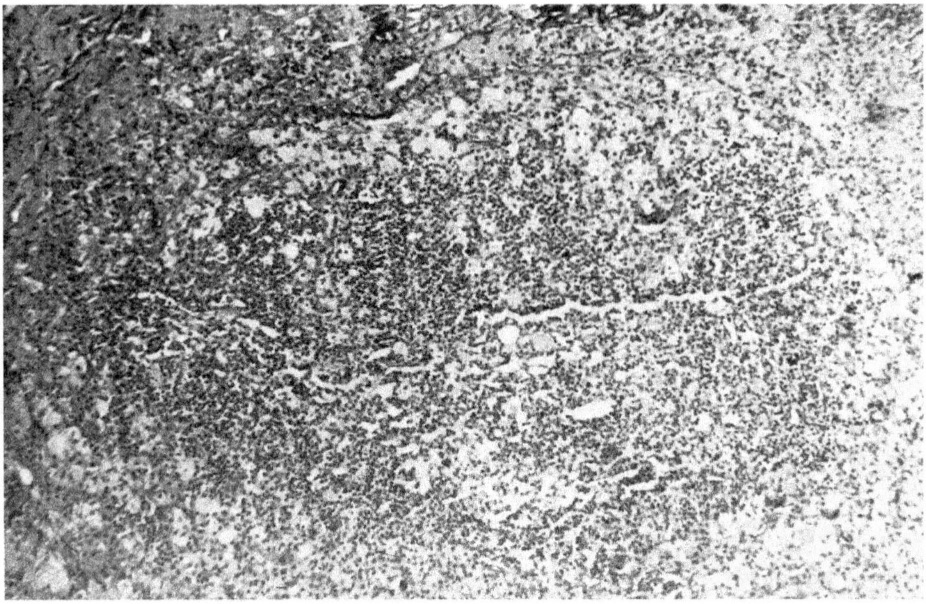

Fig. 7. Microscopic section of an overembolized kidney (Ethibloc, 0.08 ml) 2 months after embolization: Massive perirenal inflammatory reaction. HE × 60

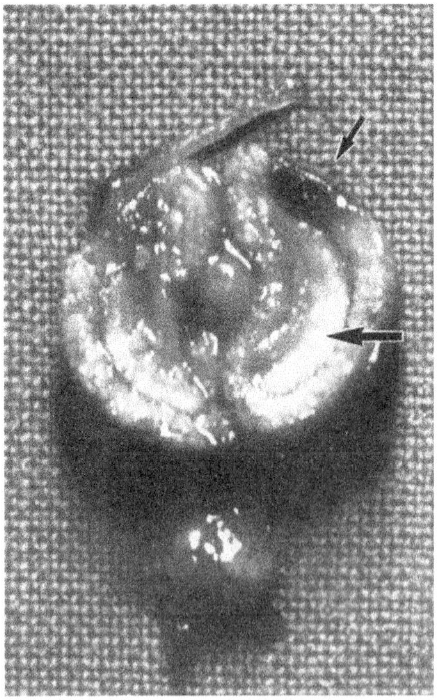

a

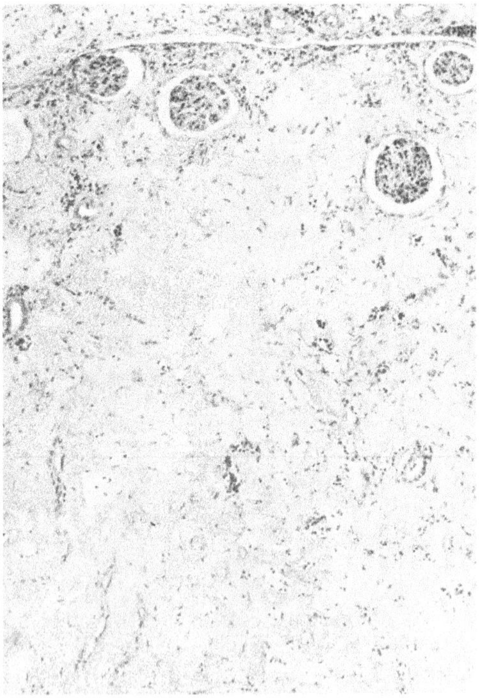

b

Fig. 8a, b. Ligation of the renal artery. **a** Cross section of the organ 2 months after ligation of the main renal artery: Intensive calcification, particularly in the medullar area (*large arrow*) with remaining parenchyma (*small arrow*). **b** Corresponding microscopic section: Note slightly collapsed glomerula in the outer renal cortex. HE × 150

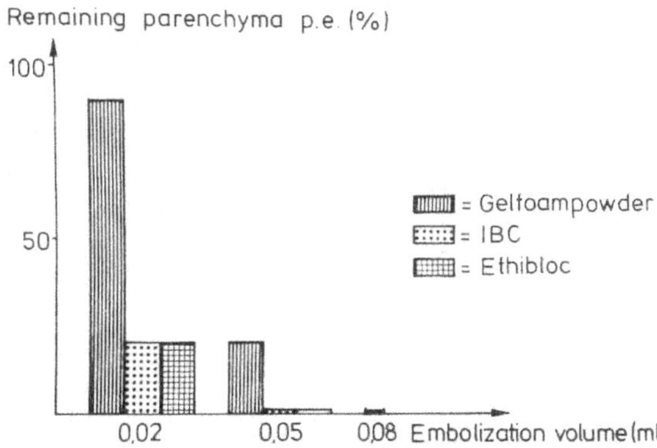

Fig. 9. Long-term results comparing the effects of Gelfoam powder, NBC, and Ethibloc in normal organs. The diagram shows the volume dependency of each embolization medium. Results are not improved from 0.05 ml to 0.07 ml, but hilar paravasation and perirenal reaction occur in 0.07 ml. Ideal embolization volume 0.05 ml (*p.e.*, post embolization)

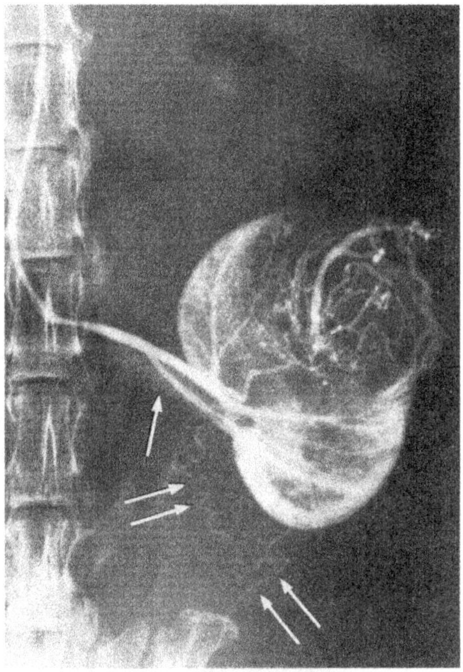

Fig. 10. Selective renal arteriography of a DMN-induced tumor of the left upper pole. Tumor vessels communicate via anastomosis with retroperitoneal collaterals (*arrow*). Note also early filling of renal vein!

Adenocarcinomas. Are well vascularized. In 35% they are nondifferentiated epithelial tumors and about 65% show tubular and papillary differentiations (Fig. 11).

Mesenchymal Tumors. Are poorly vascularized and in late stages they show increasing central fibrosis with areas of necrosis and calcification. Diffuse infiltration of the renal tissue by small spindle cells is found (Fig. 11).

In both tumor types, cysts usually filled with blood are found in the cortex and in the medulla close to the cortex. This cystic degeneration is frequently one of the first angiographic signs of tumor (*Richter* et al., 1981). Both types in later stages show sinusoidal vessels, especially in marginal areas. The different tumor

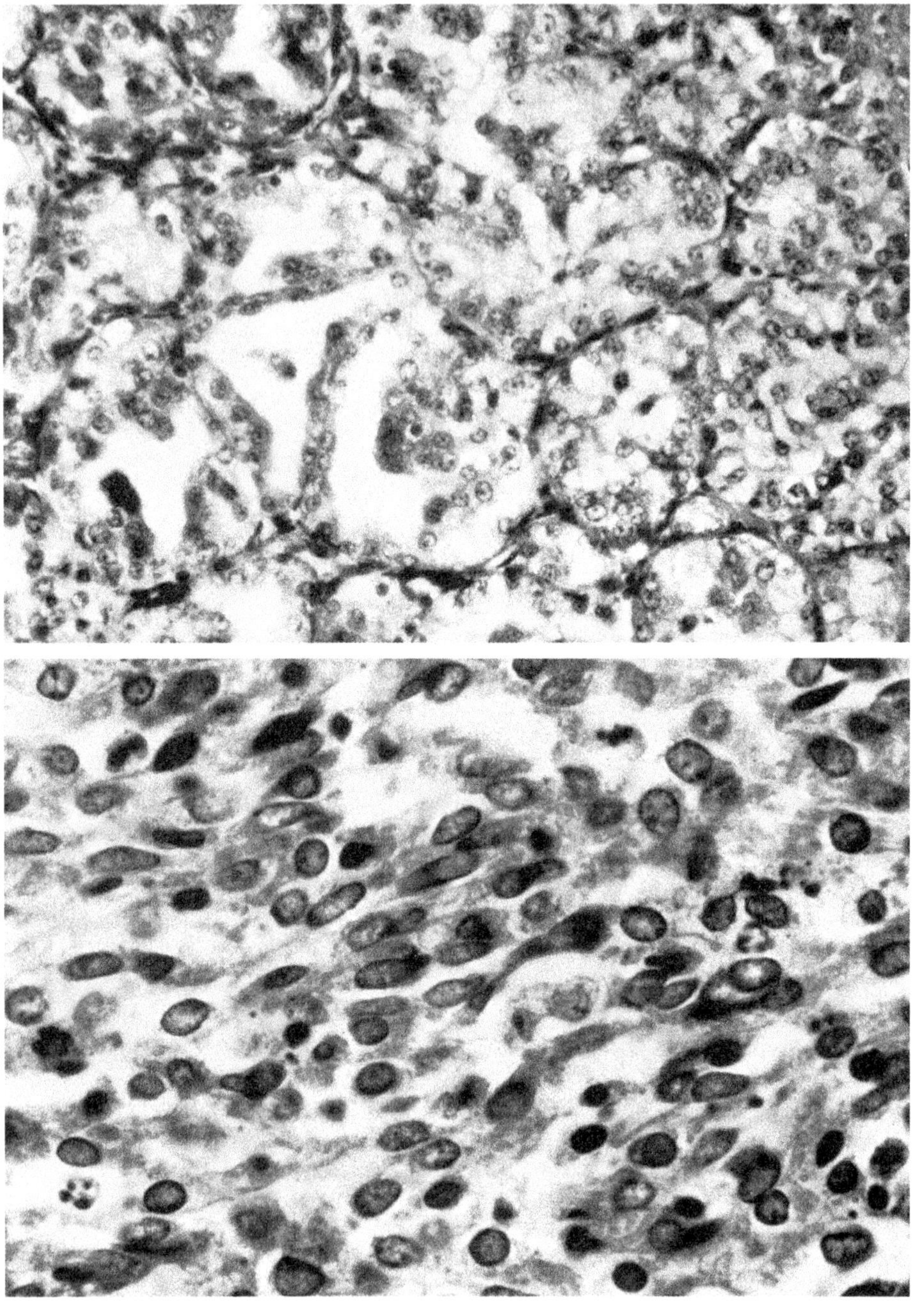

a

b

Fig. 11 a, b. Microscopic sections of main tumor types developed by DMN. **a** Adenocarcinoma with moderately differentiated tubular structures. HE×420. **b** Mesenchymal tumor predominately with spindle cells showing high hyperchromacy and moderate collaging fiber formation. EVG×420

Table 3. Relationship between TNM classification of renal tumors (*Wallace* 1974) and our classification by tumor size without exact tumor staging (i.e., liver and bone metastases)

TNM system	Classification by tumor size
$T_1N_0M_0$ $T_2N_0M_0$ $T_3N_0M_0$	M (medium size: less than 6 times volume of normal kidney)
$T_4N_0M_0$	L (large size: more than 6 times volume of normal kidney)

Table 4. Effectiveness of capillary embolization in renal rat tumors according to size of the tumor, choice of embolization medium, and complications

Embolization medium	Tumor necrosis		Complications
	M	L	
Ethibloc	83%	53%	–
IBC/Lipiodol	80%	46%	Reflux ($n=3$), Pulmonary embolism ($n=4$)
Gelfoam powder	63%	11%	Pulmonary embolism ($n=3$)
Ligation	17%	–	–

M tumors less than 6 times volume of normal kidney
L tumors more than 6 times volume of normal kidney

types are seen in all stages. As a representative parameter for tumor spread, only the lungs and perirenal tissue are examined. No lymphatic or hematogenous metastases could be detected. The pulmonary ($n=2$) and brain ($n=1$) tumors that occurred could be differentiated as primary neoplasms. The application of the TNM system (*Wallace* et al. 1975) to these tumors is less important than the fact that the contralateral not embolized renal tumor is the most limiting factor for the survival rate. Therefore no detailed tumor screening (i.e. for bone metastases) was performed. In capillary embolization, preembolic determination of the vascular volume represents the predominant problem. Tumors are classified according to their size (see above). Table 3 shows the relationship of our classification to the TNM system.

3.2.2.2 Tumor Embolization

The effectiveness of the different embolization media in correlation to tumor size and to complications is shown in Table 4.

Ethibloc. Microscopically it is found homogenously distributed within all arterial vascular compartments, including tumor sinusoids, with complete obstruction of the vascular lumen (Fig. 12). Veins are rarely reached, but only with partial occlusion. In larger tumors (L) Ethibloc is seen in central veins twice as frequently as in

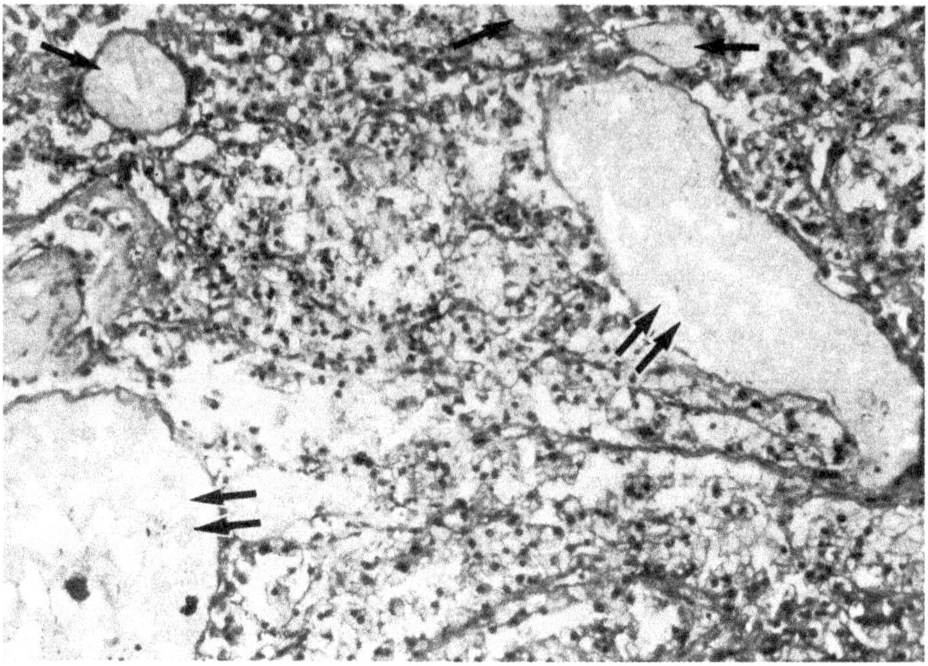

Fig. 12. Microscopic section of an adenocarcinoma occluded by Ethibloc: All arterial vessels – segmental arteries, tumor sinusoids, capillaries (*arrows*) – are completely occluded. HE × 270

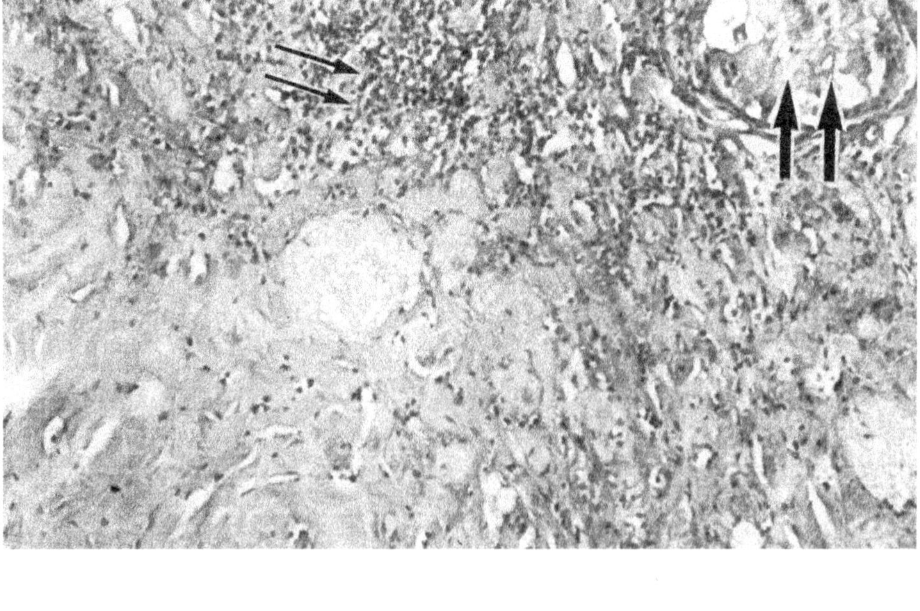

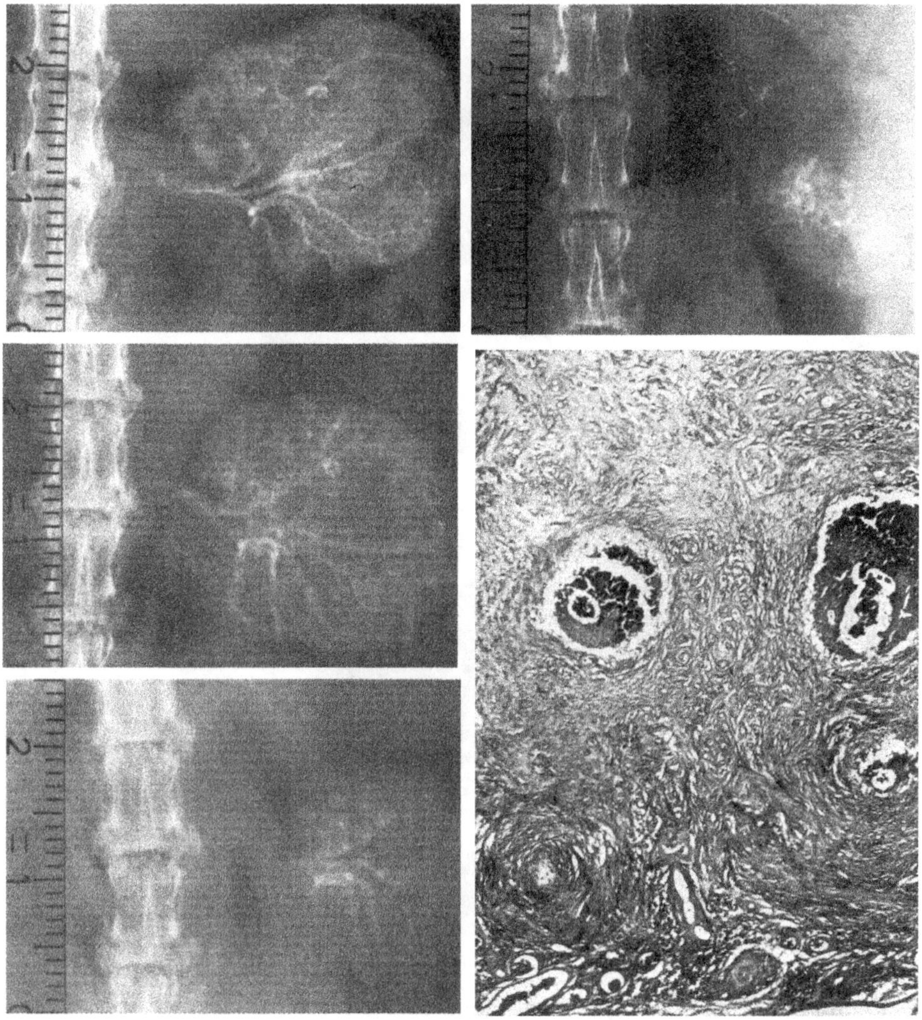

a b c d e

Fig. 14a–e. Postembolic course of a medium-sized (M) tumor following embolization with NBC/Lipiodol. **a** One week after embolization: structure of tumor vessels still visible. The size of the tumor corresponds to about 3 times the renal volume. **b** Three weeks after embolization: Incipient shrinkage of the tumor. **c** Six weeks after embolization: Remarkable shrinkage of the tumor. NBC/Lipiodol diffusely scattered in the area of the renal hilus. **d** Twelve weeks after embolization: Tumor shrinkage to one fifth of initial size. NBC residue still visible. **e** Microscopic section of the same tumor embolized 12 weeks before: Complete sclerosis of the tumor with focal inflammatory granulation tissue. Black masses within the sinusoid represent residue of NBC/Lipiodol with surrounding foreign body granulomas. EvG × 40

Fig. 13. Microscopic section of a DMN-induced tumor 2 months after Ethibloc embolization: Complete necrosis of the tumor and renal parenchyma. Slight inflammatory infiltration (*arrows*). Arteriole and tumor sinusoids still occluded by Ethibloc (*arrow*). HE × 140

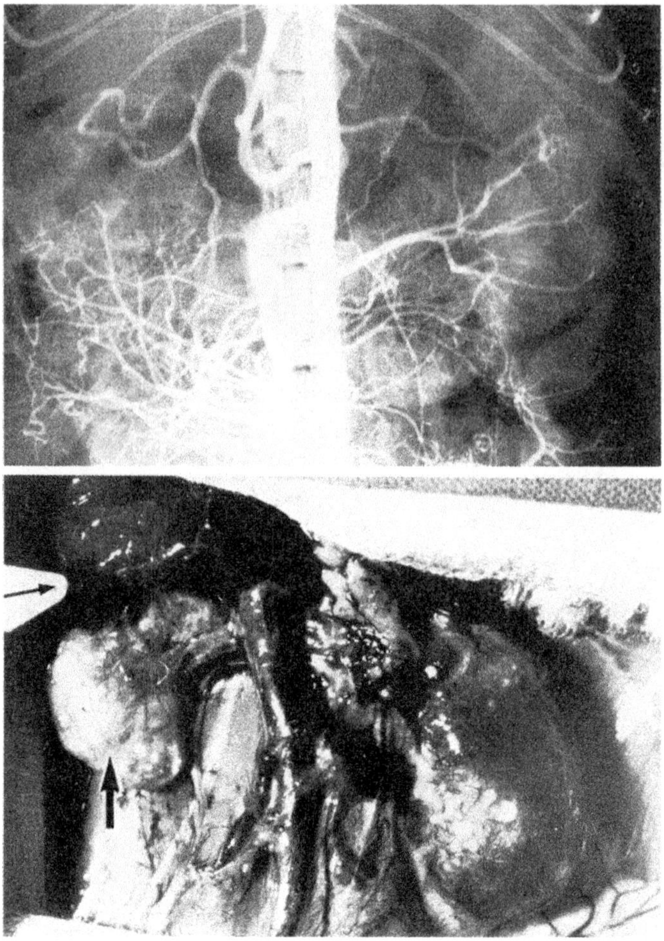

a

b

Fig. 15 a, b

medium-sized tumors (M), but no pulmonary embolism is observed. Of all medium-sized (M) tumors, 83% show total necrosis microscopically (Fig. 13). Tumors classified as $T_{1/2}$ are all necrotic. Larger tumors show complete necrosis in only 54%.

NBC/Lipiodol. Microscopically it is found in all arterial vascular compartments, including tumor sinusoids, relatively frequently also in veins [in 70% of large tumors (L)]. In four cases there was pulmonary embolism. Despite double ligation of the catheter in three animals, reflux into the aorta occurred, leading to gangrene of the left hind paw. In four cases the catheter was occluded irreversibly despite preinjection of 40% glucose. In 10% the main renal artery is recanalized. 81% of the medium-sized (M) and all $T_{1/2}$ tumors are completely necrotic and remarkably shrunken (Fig. 14). In 45% of the large tumors (L) tumor necrosis is complete.

Gelfoam Powder. Gelfoam particles are *never* documented in capillaries or tumor sinusoids microscopically, but in more than 50% of cases they are found in veins. In

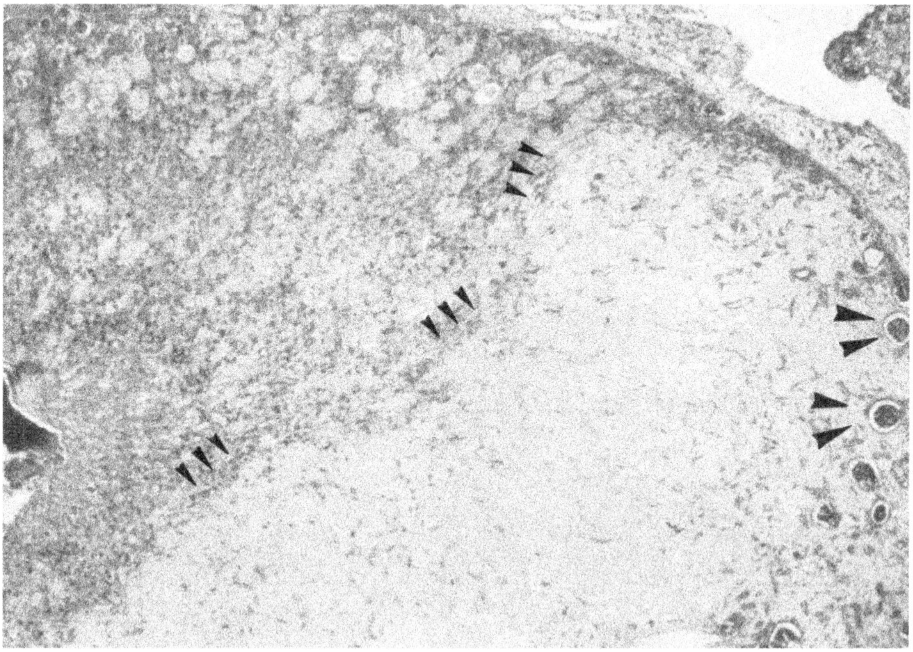

c

Fig. 15a–c. Follow-up study of a Gelfoam embolization. **a** Radiograph: 10 weeks after embolization of the right kidney: Despite occlusion of the main renal artery, recanalized tumor via anastomosis deriving from the celiac artery and hepatic artery. Note on the left vascular irregularity indicating tumor growth of contralateral kidney. **b** At necropsy, completely necrotic tumor (*large arrow*). Intact tumor tissue (*small arrow*) grown into the liver. Contralateral tumor in the meantime grown to 4 times its volume. **c** Microscopic section of the same tumor: the upper part on the left represents diffusely atrophic renal tissue whereas the right part reveals former tumor replaced by sclerosis (*small arrows*). Obviously intact glomerula are marked by big arrows. HE×30

three animals there was fatal pulmonary embolism. Microscopically, 63% of medium-sized (M) tumors are completely necrotic. In $T_{1/2}$ tumors, despite macroscopic complete tumor necrosis, areas with intact surviving tumor cells are found at microscopy in 20% (Fig. 15). In large tumors (L) total tumor necrosis is achieved in only 11%.

Ligation. Microscopically only 17% of the tumors of medium size (M) show complete necrosis. Total necrosis was *never* achieved in tumors with larger size (L). *Calcification,* which is rarely seen with the other embolization media, is *present in 74%* (Fig. 16). In 50% recurrences occur owing to intensive collaterals which are documented angiographically (Fig. 16).

3.2.3 Capillary Embolization in Canine Kidney

If the embolization procedure is performed according to the above-mentioned schedule for Ethibloc with pre- and postinjection of 40% glucose, the embolizing

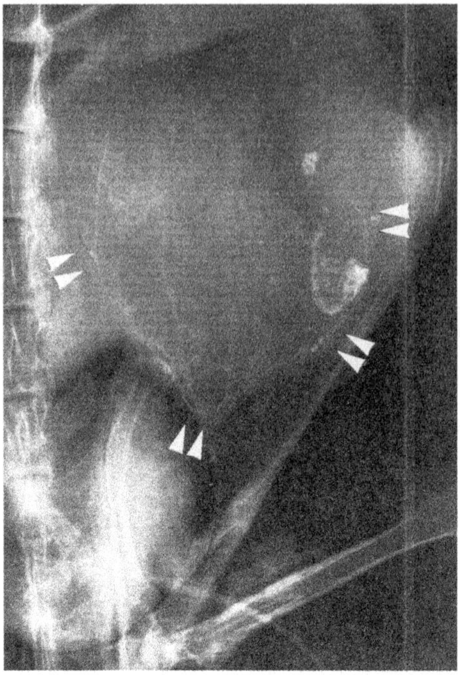

Fig. 16. Angiogram for identification of iliac collaterals 2 months after arterial ligation in a DMN-induced renal tumor: Catheter position in the left iliac artery: Numerous collaterals feed the lower part of the tumor (*arrows*). The entire tumor is outlined as a soft tissue mass. In the lateral part of the tumor, calcifications are present

a 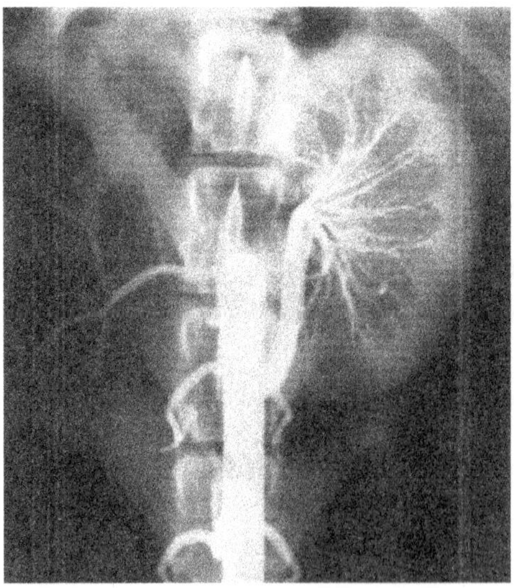

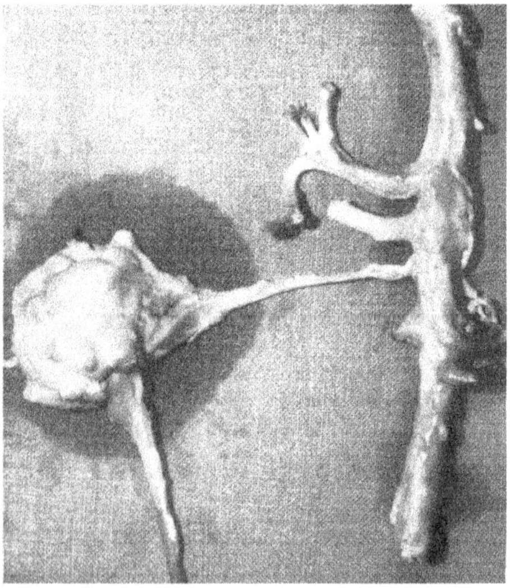 b

Fig. 17 a, b. Canine kidney embolization with Ethibloc. **a** Aortography 3 months after embolization of the right kidney. No filling of the occluded renal vessels on the right. **b** Specimen of the same kidney 3 months after embolization: Granulation tissue in the area of the renal hilus, the renal artery is still visible as a fibrotic band as well as the ureter

Table 5. General and specific demands for embolization media in tumor treatment

General conditions	Specific conditions
Biological inertness	Suitable viscosity ($\approx$ 200 cps)
No recanalization	Particle size [a] $\leqq 7\ \mu m$
Sterilizability	Radiodensity > 200 mg iodine/ml
	Controllable occlusion mechanism

[a] If no liquids are used

agent is found homogenously distributed within the arterial system and glomerular capillaries (embolization volume 4.5–5.5 ml). Three to five months later, total necrosis of the shrunken kidney (17–21 mm) is found: in three of our cases, the organ could not even be detected in the area of the renal pelvis (Fig. 17). Detailed results are described elsewhere (*Kauffmann* et al., to be published), but for clinical application the following problems are emphasized: Injection pressure rises towards the end of the embolization procedure because Ethibloc reaches the capillaries and precipitation starts. The subsequent injection leads to dilatation of the main renal arteries. Both factors support sliding back of the balloon catheter towards the aorta, thus representing a stop signal for Ethibloc injection. If the tip of the catheter still has a distance of 3 cm to the origin of the renal artery, it is quite possible to clear the catheter with a 40% glucose injection. In this case, gentle controlled glucose injection may result in a slow sliding back of the balloon catheter. If there is only a very small distance between the balloon tip and the aorta, then instead of glucose injection, quick aspiration of the Ethibloc and withdrawal of the catheter has to be performed. We observed no file formation of the precipitated Ethibloc resulting in embolic reflux.

4 Discussion

The requirements for embolization media in clinical tumor treatment are well known (Table 5). They should be biologically inert, i.e., with no local toxicity or cancerogenicity. Any tendency to recanalization is unwanted. They should not cause infections as, for example, occasionally observed in muscle fibres (*Marx* et al. 1978; *Steckenmesser* et al. 1976). If capillary embolization is aimed for, the technical requirements for embolization media (Table 5) should include that liquids are used with a suitable viscosity ($\sim$ 200 cP) and radiodensity (>200 mg iodine/ml), and that there is the possibility of regulating the occlusion mechanism.

4.1 Technical Requirements

4.1.1 Biological Inertness

Ethibloc and Gelfoam powder are inert, whereas with NBC specific perivascular inflammatory reactions and foreign-body granulomas were often found both by us and by authors (*Freeny* et al. 1979; *Günther* et al. 1978). The latter is discussed as a possible source of tumor induction, but this has never been proven (*Athanasoulis* 1980; *Gottlob* et al. 1974; *Ott* 1970).

4.1.2 Recanalization

With Gelfoam powder, there is frequently recanalization (*Berenstein* 1979; *Greenfield* 1980; *Jander* 1980; Fig. 4). Even NBC is occasionally recanalized, as it is clearly difficult to avoid enclosure of blood, this being the possible origin of recanalization. Ethibloc is never recanalized, because there is complete filling of the vascular lumen without enclosure of blood. Furthermore Ethibloc is homogenously distributed throughout the entire arterial system. This leads to complete necrosis of the embolized organ before significant resorption of the polypeptide (Zein) can take place.

4.1.3 Particle Size

As NBC/Lipiodol and Ethibloc/Glucose are injected as liquids, their ability to reach the capillaries depends on viscosity and time and type of occlusion mechanism. The particle size of Gelfoam powder (10–100 μm) is clearly too large to reach the capillaries.

4.1.4 Radiodensity

The radiodensity of an occluding agent should exceed 200 mg iodine/ml. This is necessary for monitoring of the substance in smaller arteries, to evaluate the parenchymal stain as a rough parameter of capillary distribution, and especially in presence of a.v. shunts, to detect in good time the embolization medium in the draining veins. The radiodensities of Gelfoam powder/Urografin and NBC/Lipiodol (Fig. 1) are suitable. The contrast of Ethibloc with 120 mg iodine/ml is sufficient only for its fluoroscopic verification in main arteries; parenchymal stain and early venous detection are not guaranteed. *Warning:* Addition of Lipiodol to Ethibloc in order to enhance contrast is dangerous, especially if larger amounts of the substance reach the capillary bed: Lipiodol separates from the precipitating Ethibloc and diffuses into the venous system. A preliminary incomplete study in collaboration with Ethicon (Hamburg) and Byk Gulden (Konstanz), has attempted to enhance the contrast of this embolization medium. The oleum papaveris in Ethibloc is replaced by its iodized ester, so that the quantity relation between the Zein and the oil is kept constant, and the physical conditions of the occlusion mechanism are not changed (unpublished data).

4.1.5 Viscosity

Embolization media with extremely *high* viscosity, such as silicon elastomer (*Wolf* 1978) or polyurethane foam (*Doppman* et al. 1978), entail the danger of unwanted mechanical obstruction of the catheter or of smaller arteries before the occlusion mechanism starts. Embolization media with extreme *low* viscosity, e.g., NBC/Lipiodol or methylmethacrylate (*Strecker* et al. 1979), on the other hand, facilitate venous passage, especially in the presence of a.v. shunts, because inadvertent rapid injection is possible and intravascular propagation might become so fast that the occlusion mechanism starts too late. Polymerization of NBC/Lipiodol is catalyzed by anions and the timing is strictly fixed in dependence on the proportions of the mixture (10 s for Lipiodol/NBC mixed 1 : 1). Therefore not only speed of injection but also time of polymerization determines whether the arterial or venous compartment is reached. *The fixed timing of the NBC polymerization, combined with its low viscosity, is the main reason for difficulties in handling it.*

The *ideal* viscosity of an embolization medium for capillary propagation should be so high that its further transport is limited by the rising intravascular flow resistance within the capillary bed. This is the case with Ethibloc which is only transported into the capillaries if 40% glucose is preinjected. The quantity and concentration of glucose is abruptly reduced on reaching the venous compartment, because it is diluted according to the ratio of the volumes of the arterial and venous compartments, namely 1:4 (*Boylan* et al. 1970). If glucose concentration drops, Ethibloc precipitation starts. *Therefore in glucose-regulated Ethibloc embolization, passage from the arterial to the venous compartment starts the occlusion mechanism.*

4.1.6 Passage Through Catheters

Unexpected occlusion of the angiographic tube by NBC/Lipiodol may happen even to the experienced examiner. The reason is that the NBC polymerizes even in contact with traces of aniones. Gelfoam has no such transportation problems as the definite occlusion only starts following some minutes of contact with blood by thrombus formation. In Ethibloc we never observed catheter occlusion if 40% glucose was pre-injected.

4.1.7 Pre- and Postinjection of Clearing Substances

With Gelfoam powder, pre- and postinjection to rinse the catheter is unnecessary. In NBC, only preinjection of a nonionic substance would guarantee its transport to the capillaries, avoiding obstruction of the catheter. However, using Lipiodol for preembolic rinsing might have two consequences:

1) Insufficient mixture of the pre-injected Lipiodol with the polymerization complex will result in venous propagation of the Lipiodol itself.
2) Polymerization time might be so delayed that part of the NBC/Lipiodol complex passes into the venous system.

Instead of Lipiodol, 40% glucose could be used since its high osmotic effect aggregates hydroxyl ions, facilitating capillary transport. Postinjection of 40% glucose alone proved to be impossible as the delay of polymerization is too short and the direct contact of NBC/Lipiodol and glucose leads to catheter obstruction. Therefore a small amount of Lipiodol is postinjected and this is pushed forward by the following glucose injection. On the other hand, if postembolic clearing of the catheter is not performed or is not adequate, it might stick to the intravascular cast of embolized NBC. With *Ethibloc, pre*injection of 40% glucose guarantees capillary transport and prevents occlusion of the angiographic tube (Table 3). Clearing of the catheter could easily be performed by *post*injection of 40% glucose. This is absolutely necessary in rat experiments, otherwise reflux might occur when the catheter is withdrawn.

4.2 Animal Experiments

Independently of the embolization medium used it could be shown that the capillary-type embolization is only efficient if the substance is homogenously distributed throughout the entire arterial system from the main arteries to the capillaries. This is only well achieved if the arterial volume of the vascular system to be embolized is known.

4.2.1 Normal Organs

The most important result within this group is that success of embolization is strictly dependent on the injection volume (Fig. 9). For the rat kidney this "ideal volume" is 0.05 ml. *Insufficient quantity* of embolization medium leads to incomplete occlusion and favors recanalization. Furthermore it could be shown that there is a close correlation between microscopically detectable islands of intact parenchyma and the appearance of calcification in insufficiently embolized kidneys. Therefore the conclusion has to be made that calcifications following embolization, an observation also made by other authors (*Tada* et al. 1978), are indicators of insufficient embolization. Unspecific perirenal and inflammatory reactions like lymphocytic and granulocytic infiltration are observed in *over*embolization independently of the embolization medium used. Since the catheter tip is fixed by arterial ligation and therefore prevented from sliding back, rising intraarterial pressure possibly causes vascular rupture with intraparenchymal and subcapsular extravasations. As there is a correlation between such extravasations of embolization media and inflammatory reactions, overembolization might be discussed as the cause. If the efficiency of the embolization media is compared in *optimal* volume-orientated embolization, NBC/Lipiodol and Ethibloc/glucose are superior to Gelfoam powder or ligation. Additionally, arterial ligation is followed by extreme calcifications of the organ, with intact glomerula in the renal cortex. This shows that even collaterals of normal organs are able to maintain some intrarenal blood circulation, if no capillary-type embolization is performed.

Organ necrosis following intraarterial injections of high percent alcohol has been reported by *Ekelund* (1980, personal communication). It is possible that the 60% alcohol of the Ethibloc itself produces additionally some parenchymal necrosis. However, permanent anoxia, a condition for tumor necrosis (*Tannock* and *Steel* 1969), is only achieved by mechanical obstruction of capillaries and sinusoids by the precipitated Ethibloc.

4.2.2 Dimethylnitrosamine-induced Renal Rat Tumors

Dimethylnitrosamine proved a very powerful carcinogen: It induced interstitial mesenchymal tumors and adenocarcinomas of various differentiation in almost 100%. The validity of this tumor model consists in its frequently documented parasitic vascular supply of other organs, with vessels deriving from lumbar, mesenteric, celiac, ovarian, and other origins (Fig. 10). A disadvantage of this tumor model is that the survival rate (mean 6 weeks) is limited by the growth of the contralateral untreated tumor. Therefore lymphatic or hematogenic metastases which were not observed play a less important role for survival rate.

4.3 Embolization Volume

The embolization quantity which could be standardized in normal organs is unknown in tumors with their varying vascular structure. Estimation of the correct embolization volume therefore represents one of the major limitations of our experiments in renal rat tumors: Contrast medium injections which could give more accurate information about the vascular volume are not tolerated because of an extreme sensitivity of rats carrying bilateral renal tumors. On the other hand, fluoroscopic control of the embolization procedure itself for volume monitoring would involve a high radiation exposure to the hands of the examiner. Furthermore in NBC the injection conditions are so complicated because of its rapid reaction that fluoroscopic control cannot help to perform quick variation of injection conditions. In Ethibloc the contrast is so poor that the necessary visualization of parenchymal stain is impossible.

The vascular volume therefore is just roughly estimated according to the size of the tumor. Such estimation is only valid if tumors of different sizes have comparable vascular supply, which evidently cannot be considered as a rule. The consequence is over- and more frequently under-embolization. Some improvement of experimental results could be expected if more accurate determination of the vascular volume were possible.

4.4 Intratumoral Anastomoses

One of the outstanding results of this experimental series is the retrograde filling of ovarian collaterals via intratumoral anastomoses by injection into the main renal artery. Evidently this is only achieved by capillary transported media like NBC/Lipiodol and Ethibloc/glucose. These intratumoral anastomoses support the concept of a common multilateral arterial supply of tumors. The fact that caliber fluctuations are frequent in tumors (*Kauffmann* et al. b 1980; *Wenz* et al. 1972), with no constant narrowing of vessels as in normal organs (*Kauffmann* et al. 1975), suggests that tumor sinusoids represent a primitive irregular network deriving its supply equally from several directions. In this context the importance of the so-called angiogenesis growth factor should be mentioned: Tumor cells, especially under conditions of hypoxia, release a factor which is able to transform fibroblasts into angioblasts (*Folkman* 1974). As this factor is released in several directions, the neovascularity is multilateral, forming a spongelike vessel structure.

It is possible that there are some areas in very large tumors which might be exclusively fed by parasitic vessels, especially if separated off by areas of necrosis. This would explain poor results of capillary embolization in very large tumors (Table 4).

4.5 Arteriovenous Shunts

The high rate of pulmonary embolism with *Gelfoam powder* could be explained by the fact that in tumors Gelfoam powder passes through a.v. shunts before it reaches the capillaries. As Gelfoam powder has no self-adhesive tendency, some particles may easily pass into the venous system before they are impacted within the thrombus. Since in a.v. shunts there is a low intravascular flow resistance, any liquid embolization medium reaches the shunt before the tumor sinusoids. Being relatively nonviscous, NBC/Lipiodol passes through the a.v. shunt into the veins before the time-fixed polymerization can take place.

A possible explanation for differences in effectiveness of NBC and Ethibloc (Table 4), despite comparable capillary distribution, could be that in the vicinity of such a.v. shunts NBC/Lipiodol tends to flow through the shunt and pass over into the veins with possible pulmonary embolism (Table 4), resulting in a locally under-embolized area: This local "steal" phenomenon might be an origin of tumor recurrences. This mechanism does not equally apply to Ethibloc embolization: Its high viscosity provides a slow flow through a.v. shunts, giving it more time for precipitation. In a.v. shunts the importance of the glucose-regulated embolization starting the occlusion mechanism by changing from the arterial into the venous compartment becomes much more evident: If the preinjected 40% glucose reaches an a.v. shunt, it is diluted at once, which results in acceleration of Ethibloc precipitation. If the Ethibloc is injected slowly, medium-sized a.v. shunts will be occluded and further injection of Ethibloc will be directed into tumor sinusoids. It has to be admitted, however, that in clinical embolization with large a.v. shunts, rapid Ethibloc injection might result in a too fast passage through the shunt, followed by too late and/or incomplete precipitation, with an Ethibloc embolus being torn off into the cava. Therefore in presence of a.v. shunts – even under conditions of vascular stasis – especially at the beginning of the embolization procedure, *slow injection of the substance is mandatory.*

4.6 Disadvantages of Central Type of Occlusion

Intact tumor tissue is present in 83% and 100% respectively (Table 4) if ligation of the renal artery is performed in medium or large tumors. This correlates well with results of various authors (*Bischoff* et al. 1977; *Flamm* et al. 1981; *Grosse-Vorholt* and *Zeitler* 1980; *Chuang* and *Wallace* 1980), but it underlines at the same time that the concept of tumor embolization has to be fundamentally revised: Insufficient occlusion of the tumor by central-type embolization will lead only to secondary thrombosis in the tumor periphery, favoring collateralization and recanalization and producing only hypoxia but no anoxia. At the same time this hypoxia may induce additional parasitic neovascularity by the angiogenesis factor (*Folkman* 1974). Any results talking about tumor embolization with the Gianturco-Anderson-Wallace coil do not reflect the actual possibilities of this new angiotherapeutic technique (*Chuang* and *Wallace* 1980; *Sparwasser* et al. 1979). If future clinical studies compare radiation and surgery with the effectiveness of tumor embolization, they should make it clear whether a central or homogenous capillary type of embolization has been performed.

Another negative aspect of the central type of embolization caused by recanalization is the so-called tourniquet syndrome observed in muscle fibre embolization: Necrotic material together with metabolites like pyruvate and lactate enters the blood circulation via recanalized vessels, causing cardiac failure, hypotension, shock, and renal failure (*Kösters* and *Holzki* 1981). Though it has not been clarified whether the muscle itself or hypoxia and acidosis with release of metabolic products induces this clinical picture, the confrontation of the body with a large quantity of necrotic material has to be seriously taken into account. The capillary-type embolization using Ethibloc, having no tendency for recanalization, should prevent this. The completely anoxic organ will be surrounded by granulation tissue (Fig. 6) which provides slow resorption of metabolic products.

At present there are only two embolization media with capillary propagation in use: NBC/Lipiodol and Ethibloc/glucose. In our rat experiments the complication rate of NBC/Lipiodol includes – besides venous embolization – the reflux into the aorta despite double arterial ligation of the catheter. That this could happen despite considerable experience with this substance by the same research group underlines the problems in management of the substance in vitro and in vivo. We feel therefore that NBC/Lipiodol cannot be recommended as a capillary embolization medium fulfilling safety criteria.

4.7 Balloon-Tipped Catheters

Vascular stasis is one of the prerequisites for Ethibloc embolization. Three decisive arguments support the necessity of vascular stasis:

1) The incalculable hemodynamic situation in a.v. shunts will be diminished.
2) The effect of glucose-regulated Ethibloc injection is only established in vascular stasis.
3) Unlike other well-known embolization procedures, reflux towards the end of the procedure is safely avoided (*Greenfield* et al. 1978; *Kauffmann* et al. 1978).

Our *experiments with dogs* showed that the capillary-type embolization is possible if arterial occlusion is performed by balloon-tipped catheters instead of arterial ligation. The outstanding features of capillary-type embolization using balloon catheters are:

1) The required intraarterial pressure during Ethibloc injection for capillary transportation is well maintained. Sometimes inflation of the balloon till beginning oval distortion might be necessary.
2) The middle part of the procedure might be performed somewhat faster, especially if in clinical embolization large amounts of Ethibloc are needed (reduction of radiation exposure).
3) Towards the end of the embolization procedure when the main arteries are filled up with Ethibloc, they will be dilatated and further injection will cause the balloon to slide back.
4) If the injection speed is then reduced and subtle fluoroscopic control provided, the sliding back should be controllable.
5) In clinical embolization, arteriosclerotic plaques might cause uncalculable movements of the balloon catheter. Therefore it might be advisable to reduce the volume of the balloon at the end of the procedure so that it regains its circular shape to permit gentle and controlled sliding back.

It is easier to maintain a very slow speed by using 1-ml syringes. We prefer them to larger syringes in order to reduce the manual pressure necessary to overcome intraluminal resistance. With this controlled subtle dosage the sliding back of the balloon-tipped catheter might even be used to fill capsular branches arising close to the aorta.

As mentioned in Sect. 4.1.7, postembolic rinsing of the catheter with 40% glucose should be performed to avoid reflux of Ethibloc. When the tip of the balloon is very close to the aorta, postembolic glucose injection is not possible. In this critical situation three steps are advisable:

1) Quick aspiration of Ethibloc to separate it from its intravascular cast
2) Slow deflation of the balloon to guarantee complete precipitation
3) Slow withdrawal of the catheter

The added oleum papaveris guarantees easy tearing off of the precipitated Ethibloc without file formation at the tip of the catheter. Intraaortal blood pressure pushes the Ethibloc cast a few millimeters downstream within the renal artery.

4.8 Conclusions

1) *Central types of occlusion* as performed with the Gianturco-Andersson-Wallace coil or by ligation cannot achieve complete necrosis of normal organs and are insufficient for tumor embolization. In tumor embolization, the only indication we see for central types of occlusion is in superselective occlusion of large a.v. shunts to permit glucose-regulated Ethibloc embolization as a second step.
2) The *"peripheral" transport* of embolization media represented by Gelfoam powder reaching only the arterioles is not as effective as media transported by capillaries in normal organs and ineffective in tumor embolization.
3) Only *primary occlusion* from the *capillaries* to the main arteries by an embolization medium like Ethibloc/glucose presents some real progress in tumor embolization. Success is strictly quantity-dependent: An effort should be made to determine the vascular volume before embolization. In the future, the difficulties of performing a volume-correct embolization will present major problems.
4) Difficulties with handling and the *complication rate of NBC/Lipiodol*, i.e., pulmonary embolism, precludes its safe use in clinical embolization.
5) Small and medium-sized *arteriovenous shunts* in renal cell carcinoma will not present a contraindication for Ethibloc glucose embolization. However, care has to be taken that not too much Ethibloc reaches the venous sysem too rapidly, as little is known about possible tearing off of larger Ethibloc quantities. In this context the poor contrast of Ethibloc presents a major limiting factor for early detection of venous propagation (although contrast enhanced Ethibloc is in preparation).
6) Though results with Ethibloc are encouraging, the *recurrence rate* in very large tumors shows limitations in effectiveness of capillary embolization too.

We suggest the following definition of occlusion types:

Central type: large arteries, large a.v. shunts (coil, detachable balloon)

Peripheral type: smaller vessels, i.e., visceral bleeding (0.5–1 mm diameter Gelfoam particles)

Capillary type: Primary occlusion of the entire arterial system including the capillaries, i.e., tumor embolization (Ethibloc/glucose)

The results should encourage the clinical use of Ethibloc/glucose. The capillary-type embolization is recommended particularly for palliative tumor treatment and a.v. malformations as well as for organ-ablating embolization, for example as ultimate therapy in malignant hypertension (review in *Powischer* et al. 1980).

References

Athanasoulis CHA (1980) Therapeutic applications of angiography I. N Engl J Med 302: 1117–1125

Berenstein A, Kricheff I (1979) Catheter and material selection for transarterial embolization. Technical considerations. Part I Catheters: Radiology 132:619–630; Part II Materials: Radiology 132:631–639

Bischoff W, Thomas C, Elsässer E, Schnitzer A (1977) Wachstumsbeeinflussung experimenteller Nephroblastome durch Nierenarterienokklusion. Radiologe 17:503–508

Boylan JW, Deetjen P, Kramer W (1970) Niere und Wasserhaushalt. Urban & Schwarzenberg, München

Bücheler E, Hupe W, Klosterhalfen H, Altenaehr E, Erbe W (1978) Neue Substanz zur therapeutischen Embolisation von Nierentumoren. Fortschr. Roentgenstr 128:599–603

Chuang VP, Wallace S (1980) Current status of transcatheter management of neoplasms. Cardiovasc Intervent Radiol 3:256–267

Cromwell LD, Kerber CHW (1979) Modification of cyanoacrylate for therapeutic embolization: preliminary experience. AJR 132:799–801

Doppman JL, Aven W, Bowman RL, Wood LL, Girton H (1978) A rapidly polymerizing polyurethane for transcatheter embolization. Cardiovasc Radiol 1:109–116

Dotter CH, Goldman ML, Rösch J (1975) Instant selective arterial occlusion with isobutyl-2-cyanoacrylate. Radiology 114:227–230

Flamm J, Burkert S, Grof F (1981) Zur Problematik der transfemoralen Katheterembolisation von Nierentumoren. Aktuel Urol 12:19–22

Folkman J (1974) Tumor angiogenesis. Adv Cancer Res 19:331–338

Freeny PC, Mennemeyer R, Kidd CR, Bush WH (1979) Long-term radiographic-pathologic follow-up of patients treated with visceral transcatheter occlusion using isobutyl-2-cyanoacrylate (Bucrylate). Radiology 132:51–60

Gottlob R, Reimitzer P, Funovic J (1974) Untersuchungen zur Histotoxizität mehrerer Homologe von Zyanoakrylat-Gewebeklebern. Zentralbl Chir 99:225–227

Greenfield AJ, Athanasoulis CH, Waltmann AC, Le Moure ER (1978) Transcatheter embolization: prevention of embolic reflux – using balloon catheters. AJR 131:651–655

Greenfield AJ (1980) Transcatheter vessel occlusion: selection of methods and materials. Cardiovasc Intervent Radiol 3:222–228

Grosse-Vorholt R, Zeitler E (1980) Ergebnisse und technische Probleme der therapeutischen Gefäßembolisation unter besonderer Berücksichtigung der Spiralembolisation. Radiologe 20:188–195

Günther R, Schubert U, Bohl J, Georgi M, Marberger M (1978) Transcatheter embolization of the kidney with butyl-2-cyanoacrylate. Experimental and clinical results. Cardiovasc Radiol 1:101–108

Hard GC, Butler WH (1971a) Ultrastructural analysis of renal mesenchymal tumor induced in the rat by dimethylnitrosamine. Cancer Res 31:348–365

Hard GC, Butler WH (1971b) Ultrastructural aspects of renal adenocarcinoma induced in the rat by dimethylnitrosamine. Cancer Res 31:366–372

Hard GC, Butler WH (1971c) Morphogenesis of epithelial neoplasms induced in the rat kidney by dimethylnitrosamine. Cancer Res 31:1496–1505

Jander HP, Russinovich NA (1980) Transcatheter gelfoam embolization in abdominal, retroperitoneal, and pelvic hemorrhage. Radiology 136:337–344

Kauffmann GW, Bischoff W, Lohss B (1975) Angiomorphometrie bei malignen Tumoren. Röntgenberichte 4:271–278

Kauffmann GW, Bischoff W, Wimmer B, Roth FJ (1978) Die Wichtigkeit experimenteller Arterienverschlüsse unter besonderer Berücksichtigung ihrer Komplikationen. Fortschr. Roentgenstr 125:445–452

Kauffmann GW, Mathias K, Waldmann D (1979) Die Embolisationsbehandlung der Magen-Darm-Blutung – eine Alternative zur chirurgischen Intervention? Chirurg 50:701–703

Kauffmann GW, Wimmer B, Rohrbach R, Sommerkamp H, Kröpelin T (1980a) Nierenembolisation, Renozystographie und perkutane Nephrostomie. Radiologe 20:308–318

Kauffmann GW, Strecker EP, Bammert J, Meyer P, Wenz W (1980b) Angiomorphometry in malignant tumors and inflammatory disease. Invest Radiol 15:475–480

Kauffmann GW, Rassweiler J, Richter G, Hauenstein KH, Rohrbach R, Friedburg H (1981) Capillary embolization by ethibloc: new embolization concept tested in dog kidney. AJR 137:1163–1168

Kösters S, Holzki B (1981) Protrahiertes Tourniquet-Syndrom nach Nierenembolisation. Z Urol Nephrol 74:181–186

Magee PN, Barnes JM (1962) Induction of kidney tumors in the rat with dimethylnitrosamine (N-nitrosodimethylnitrosamine). J Pathol Bacteriol 84:19–31

Marx FJ, Eisenberger F, Bassermann R (1978) Komplikationen nach transfemoraler Nierentumorembolisation. Urologe A 17:79–84

Murphy GP, Mitrand EA, Johnston GS, Schmidt JB, Scott WW (1966) Renal tumors induced by a single dose of dimethylnitrosamine. Invest Urol 4:39–56

Ott G (1970) Fremdkörpersarkome. Exp Med Pathol Klin 32:47

Powischer G, Wolf A, Syre G (1980) Kidney embolization with collagen flocks in malignant renal hypertension. In: Anacker H, Gulotta U, Rupp N (eds) Percutaneous biopsy and therapy vascular occlusion, Int. Symp. München. Thieme, Stuttgart New York, pp 169–172

Rassweiler J, Kauffmann GW, Rohrbach R, Richter G (1980) Kapilläre Embolisation I. Verschluß des gesamten arteriellen Gefäßsystems der gesunden Rattenniere. Fortschr. Roentgenstr 133:644–653

Richter G, Rohrbach R, Kauffmann GW, Rassweiler J (1981) Kapilläre Embolisation II. Embolisation experimentell erzeugter Nierentumoren. Fortschr Roentgenstr 135:85–97

Rösch J, Dotter CT, Brown MJ (1972) Selective arterial embolization: a new method for control of acute gastrointestinl bleeding. Radiology 102:303–306

Sparwasser H, Lampante K, Deschum W, Habighorst LV, de Leon F (1979) Nierenarterienverschluß durch Spiralembolisation nach Gianturco. Aktuel Urol 10:145–152

Steckenmesser R, Bayindir S, Rothauge CF, Nöske K, Weidner W (1976): Embolisation maligner Nierentumoren. Fortschr Roentgenstr 125:251–257

Strecker EP, Kauffmann GW, Gilsbach J, Bischoff W, Wenz W (1979) Indikation und Wert der Katheterverschlußbehandlung. Fortschr Roentgenstr 131:520–528

Tada S, Sekiga R, Kino M, Shintany Y, Havada, J, Nanjoh M, Machida T, Masuda F, Miki M, Shoj R (1978) Labelled gelfoam in transcatheter arterial embolization of renal cell carcinoma. Radiology 128:825–826

Tannock F, Steel GG (1969) Quantitative techniques with study of the anatomy and function of small blood vessels in tumors. J Natl Cancer Inst 42:771–782

Thelen M, Brühl P, Gerlach F, Biersack HJ (1976) Katheterembolisation von metastasierten Nierenkarzinomen mit Butyl-2-cyanoacrylat. Fortschr Roentgenstr 124:232–235

Wallace DM, Chisholm GD, Hendry WF (1975) TMN classification for urological tumors (U.I.C.C.) 1974. Br J Urol 47:1–12

Wenz W, van Kaick G, Beduhn D, Roth FJ (1972) Abdominale Angiographie. Springer, Berlin Heidelberg New York

WHO (1976) Pathology of tumors in laboratory animals. Tumors of the rat. IARC I/2

Wolf KJ (1978) Therapeutische Embolisation von Organarterien – tierexperimentelle Untersuchungen, erste klinische Erfahrungen, Einführung eines neuen Embolisationsmaterials I. Fortschr Roentgenstr 128:414–422

Electric Transcatheter Vascular Obliteration: Electrothrombosis, Electrolysis or Electrocoagulation

F. Brunelle[1]

1 Introduction

Vessel occlusion is now a classic tool of 'interventional' radiology and many occlusive agents are used (*Kunstlinger* 1981), all of which are known to have some side-effects. One side-effect, which is common to all, is the possible embolization of non-target arteries. Moreover, embolization may be impossible when the blood flow is slowed down or stopped. Thus, the possibility of inducing an in situ thrombosis without any foreign material seemed a natural alternative.

Sawyer (1953) showed that it was possible to induce thrombosis in a vessel by passing a current across its wall. Then, *Salazar* (1961) using a Teflon-coated electrode was able to produce coronary artery thrombosis in the intact canine chest.

Nowadays, two different currents are used: direct (DC) and alternating current (AC). The mechanism of vascular obliteration differs according to the method used, and they will therefore be discussed separately.

1 Service de Radio-Pédiatrie, Hôpital Bicêtre, 78, rue de Général Leclerc, F-94270 Le Kremlin Bicetre

2 Occlusion Induced by Direct Current

2.1 Material

The DC technique uses a endovascular positive electrode, which is usually a modified guide-wire. This is introduced into the target artery through a catheter using the Seldinger technique. The tip of the electrode can be modified in several ways:

The simplest method is only a standard Teflon coated guide-wire, from which the Teflon coating at the tip has been removed (*Piton* et al. 1978; *Salazar* 1961; *Thompson WA* et al. 1977, 1979; *Thompson* et al. 1979); however, platinum electrodes have been used by several investigators (*Piton* et al. 1978; *Thompson WA* et al. 1979). A large dispersive electrode (bovine ground-plate) placed under the patient or around the animal leg is used as the negative electrode and the current is delivered by a DC power supply.

2.2 In Vitro Experiments

In vitro experiments showed that passing DC through a pair of electrodes placed in heparinized blood produces a clot, the size of which is approximately proportional to the amount (in Coulombs) of current (*Piton* et al. 1978; *Sawyer* and *Pate* 1953). The current used varies from 2 to 10 mA with a voltage varying from 10 to 50 V.

2.3 In Vivo Experiments

Direct current electrothrombosis was used to occlude splanchnic arteries and surgically constructed arteriovenous fistulas as well as to control induced splenic haemorrhage in dogs (*Phillips* 1973; *Thompson* et al. 1977, 1979; *Thompson WA* et al. 1979; *Tragarth* et al. 1976).

Several groups have used this technique (*Piton* et al. 1978; *Salazar* 1961) to occlude small arteries in man unsuitable for embolization or to permanently occlude the trunk of embolized vessels. These experiments and initial clinical results have shown that the occlusion obtained is permanent.

Nevertheless several disadvantages and problems are encountered with this method, namely:

A time of up to 1 h is needed to occlude large vessels.

Electrolysis of the tip of the electrode may occur because of the long time needed for thrombosis.

There is a possibility of distal embolization due to fragmentation of the clot produced around the electrode.

The technique is not consistent (*Piton* et al. 1978; *Salazar* 1961; *Thompson WA* et al. 1979).

3 Occlusion Induced by Alternating Current

Gold was the first to use AC in man, to occlude a pseudo-aneurysm in the head of the pancreas (*Gold* et al. 1975). Previous studies in animals (*Phillips* 1973) using AC encountered major obstacles:

The amount of current necessary to coagulate the blood vessel differed only slightly from the amount of current which caused rupture.
Adherence of the electrode to the vessel wall occurred frequently.

In *Phillips'* experiment, the positive electrode is a guide-wire and the negative electrode is a Bovie ground-plate.

The impedance of this unipolar system is highly variable (*Dobbie* 1969; *Thompson WA* et al. 1979; *Tragarth* et al. 1976). We believe that this is due to many variables, including variation in the length of the electrode and variation in the area of contact between the patient's skin and the ground-plate. This variation in the impedance of the unipolar electrode system may explain the difficulties in accurately controlling the amount of current to be delivered. It has been showed that a bipolar electrode may be more effective than a unipolar one in electrocoagulation of the bleeding canine stomach. Moreover, the lesion seems to be more localized (*Moore* et al. 1978).

We then developed a bipolar electrode to overcome these difficulties.

3.1 The Bipolar Electrode

A straight Teflon guide-wire (o.d. 0.88 mm) with the central core removed, is used as the outer part of the electrode (*Brunelle* et al. 1980).

The Teflon coating is stripped from the last 5 mm of the guide-wire and a thin stainless steel wire (0.15 mm diameter) is then insulated along its entire length with a small Teflon tube (i.d. 0.2 mm, o.d. 0.4 mm). A copper bead is then welded to the tip and a larger Teflon tube is slid over the insulated wire up to the copper bead. The insulated inner wire is then slid inside the lumen of the outer guide-wire. The distal part of the electrode is composed of three different parts: the distal copper bead welded to the inner wire, the large Teflon tube insulating the copper bead and the last 5 mm of the outer guide-wire, from which the Teflon has been removed. The proximal part of the outer guide-wire is uncoiled and connected to an electric plug; the inner wire is directly connected to another electric plug. The proximal end of the electrode is glued to prevent dismantling (Fig. 1).

3.2 Electrocoagulation Unit

We used a surgical electrocoagulation unit as the AC generator. This generator includes a system to monitor the exact voltage and amperage of the current and the time of application. Small arteries were obliterated in dogs, with occlusion being obtained in less than 30 s (*Brunelle* et al. 1979). This method is safe and reliable

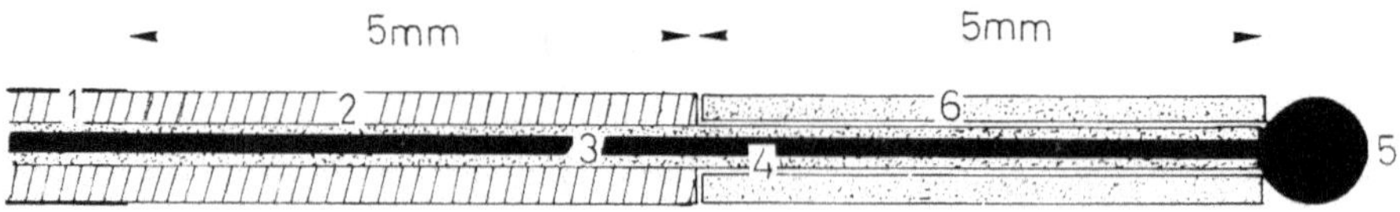

Fig. 1. *1,* 0.88 mm Teflon coated guide-wire[1]; *2,* Part of the guide-wire (electrode neutral part from which Teflon has been removed); *3,* Central core (diameter: 0.15 mm); *4,* Inner Teflon tube (I.D.: 0.2 mm; O.D.: 0.4 mm)[1]; *5,* distal copper bead (active part); *6,* Outer Teflon tube (I.D.: 0.6 mm; O.D.: 0.8 mm)[1]

and no complications were observed. We are currently studying the follow-up of the occlusions. Preliminary results indicate that AC electrocoagulation leads to hyalinization of the vessel wall, intimal burn and subsequent thrombosis. Such a thrombosis is thought to be permanent, but more experiments are needed.

4 Discussion

Two types of electrically induced vascular occlusion are used ar present. The advantages of these two methods over classic embolization are that no foreign material is used and that there is no risk of non-target vessel embolization.

Direct current vessel obliteration has some drawbacks. These are the long time necessary to induce occlusion, the possibility of electrolysis of the tip of the electrode, the possibility of distal embolization, the inconsistency of the method and the possibility of dermal burn at the site of the ground-plate.

Alternating current obliteration with a bipolar electrode alleviates all these difficulties. Nevertheless, the mechanism of occlusion is still uncompletely understood.

4.1 Direct Current Obliteration

It has been said that occlusion is mainly due to reversion of the normal polarity of the vessel wall. Then, platelets are attracted to the vessel wall and to the electrode, leading to localized thrombosis (*Sawyer* 1953).

Samuelsson et al. (1980) showed that it was possible to destroy the lung in the rabbit by electrolysis. This method is essentially the same as DC electrocoagulation, but the positive electrode is placed in the lung instead of in the vessels. They showed that there is no significant rise in temperature around the electrode and that there is a liberation of chlorine ions with a drop of pH around the positive electrode. Chlorine destroys surrounding tissues probably by its oxydizing effect. Thus, if platelet attraction is responsible for local thrombosis, liberation of chlorine may lead to thrombosis by protein denaturation. Direct current vascular occlusion should therefore be called either endovascular electrolysis or endovascular electrothrombosis.

1 Laboratoires Ingenor, 70, rue Orfila, F-75020 Paris

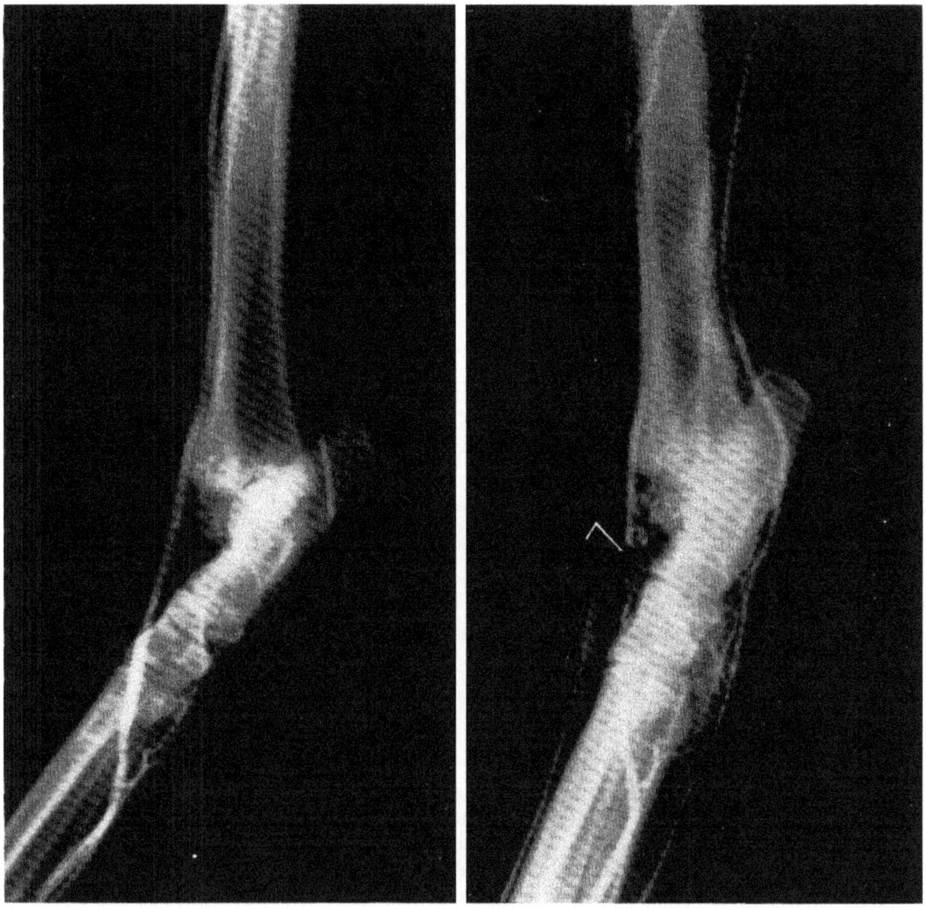

a b

Fig. 2. **a** Angiogram of right anterior tibial artery before electrocoagulation. **b** Right anterior tibial angiogram. Four weeks after electrocoagulation there is a complete occlusion of the anterior tibial artery (*arrow*) with some collateral flow through peri-articular arteries

4.2 Alternating Current Electrocoagulation

It has been shown that in AC-induced coagulation the injury is due to local rise in temperature leading to coagulation of surrounding tissues (*Brown* 1977; *Burton* 1976–77; *Dobbie* 1969; *Geddes* et al. 1977; *Organ* 1977–77; *Siegel* and *Dunn* 1965). Thrombosis is then a secondary phenomenon due to alteration of the vessel wall (*Anderson* et al. 1978). In this case, because of the vessel wall lesion, thrombosis should be permanent. Then the term of endovascular electrocoagulation should be reserved for AC-induced endovascular occlusion. Fig. 2a, b shows the right anterior tibial artery before and after electrocoagulation.

5 Conclusions

Electrocoagulation and electrothrombosis are two very effective ways of occluding vessels. They are safe, reliable and, because they do not use any foreign material, there is no risk of non-target vessel embolization.

6 Summary

The different techniques for inducing a vascular occlusion using an endovascular electrode and an electric source are described. Two main techniques are available at present, these use either a direct current (DC) or an alternating current (AC). Occlusion with the DC technique is probably due to platelet attraction to the endovascular electrode and to blood electrolysis, leading to endovascular liberation of chlorine. Some disadvantages are inherent in this method, one being the long time necessary to obtain occlusion. With the AC technique using a bipolar electrode, the occlusion is due to local rise in temperature. Occlusion is obtained in less than 60 s. These two techniques have major advantages over classic embolization and will be certainly developed in the future.

References

Anderson JH, Kaufman HH, Woo J, Handel SF (1978) Transcatheter technique for producing intimal trauma for a canine vascular occlusion model. AJR 130:793–794

Brunelle F, Kunstlinger F, Suillard J, Roche A, Doyon D (1979) Electro-coagulation endovasculaire expérimentale. Utilisation d'un courant alternatif et d'une electrode bipolaire (étude préliminaire). J Radiol 60:129–132

Brunelle F, Kunstlinger F, Doyon D (1980) A bipolar electrode for vascular electro-coagulation with alternating current. Radiology 137:239–240

Brown BH, Johnson SG, Betts RP, Henry L (1977) Burns thresholds to radio frequency leakage currents from surgical diathermy equipment. J Med Eng Technol 9:277–281

Burton CV (1976–77) RF lesion generation. Appl Neurophysiol 39:77–79

Dobbie AK (1969) The electrical aspects of surgical diathermy. Biomed Eng 4–5:206–216

Geddes LA, Silva LF, Deloitt DP, Pearce JA (1977) What's new in electrosurgical instrumentation. Med Instrum 11:355–361

Gold RE, Blair DC, Finlay JB, Johnston WB (1975) Transarterial electrocoagulation therapy of a pseudo-aneurysm in the head of the pancreas. AJR 125:422–426

Hilal SK, Michelsen JW, Driller J, Leonard E (1974) Magnetically guided devices for vascular exploration and treatment. Radiology 113:529–540

Hirschfeld BJ, Clark HC, Thompson WM (1980) The effect of temperature and pH in transcatheter electro-coagulation [abstr]. Invest Radiol 15:402

Kunstlinger F, Brunelle F, Chaumont P, Doyon D (1981) Review. Vascular occlusive agents. AJR 136:151–156

McAlister DS, Johnsrude I, Miller MM, Clapp J, Thompson WM (1979) Occlusion of acquired renal arteriovenous fistula with transcatheter electrocoagulation. AJR 132: 998–1000

Moore JP, Silvis SE, Vennes JA (1978) Evaluation of bipolar electro-coagulation in canine stomachs. Gastrointest Endosc 24:148–151

Organ LW (1976–77) Electro-physiologic principles of radiofrequency lesion making. Appl Neurophysiol 39: 69–76
Phillips JF (1973) Transcatheter electro-coagulation of blood vessels. Invest Radiol 8: 295–304
Phillips JF, Robinson AE, Johnsrude I, Jackson DC (1975) Experimental closure of arteriovenous fistula by transcatheter electro-coagulation. Radiology 115: 319–321
Piton J, Billerey J, Renou AM, Constant P, Caille JM (1978) Vascular thrombosis induced by direct electric current. Neuroradiology 16: 385–388
Salazar AE (1961) Experimental myocardial infarction. Induction of coronary thrombosis in the intact closed-chest dog. Circ Res 9: 1351
Samuelsson L, Olin T, Berg NO (1980) Electrolytic destruction of lung tissue in the rabbit. Acta Radiol [Diag] (Stockh) 21: 447–454
Sawyer PN, Pate JW (1953) Bio-electric phenomena as an etiologic factor in intravascular thrombosis. Am J Physiol 175: 103–107
Sigel B, Dunn MR (1965) The mecanism of blood vessel closure by high frequency electrocoagulation. SGO 121: 823–831
Taren JA, Gabrielsen TO (1970) Radiofrequency thrombosis of vascular malformations with a transvascular magnetic catheter. Science 168: 138–141
Thompson WM, Johnsrude I, Jackson DC, McAlister S, Miller MD, Pizzo SV (1979) Vessel occlusion with transcatheter electro-coagulation: initial clinical experience. Radiology 133: 335–340
Thompson WM, Pizzo SV, Jackson DC, Johnsrude I (1977) Transcatheter electrocoagulation. A therapeutic angiographic technique for vessel occlusion. Invest Radiol 12: 146–153
Thompson WA, McAlister DS, Miller M, Pizzo SV, Jackon DC, Johnsrude I (1979) Transcatheter electro-coagulation experimental evaluation of the anode. Invest Radiol 14: 41–47
Tragarth B, Lynch PR, Kang TH (1976) Intravascular electrically induced thrombosis in the dog. Radiology 121: 55–57
Uylings JHM, Himbergen AV (1978) Safety precautions in electrosurgery. Medica Mundi 23: 116–121

Manufacturing-Derived Impurities in Angiography

V. Hegedüs, O. Winding, J. Grønvall, and P. Faarup[1]

1 Introduction

The aim of this report is to summarise results on thrombo-embolic damage caused by involuntary iatrogenic introduction of manufacturing impurities into arteries during the angiographic procedure. Subsequently the biological significance and consequences of such foreign body embolisation will be discussed.

The terms thrombosis and embolus were introduced by *Virchow* (1856). He also investigated experimentally the biological significance of foreign bodies injected into the vascular bed and stated that arterial occlusion might occasionally be the cause of gangrene. Further investigations made by *Panum* confirmed that vascular obstruction can be caused by thrombi or by 'solid particles introduced' (1862).

In 1963 *Garvan* and *Gunnar* demonstrated that infusion solutions are contaminated with large amounts of both organic and inorganic particles ranging in size from very small to 100 µm. They also demonstrated (1964) that these sterile particles are produced during the manufacture of the infusion solution. The same authors investigated lungs from patients previously treated with large quantities of

1 Department of Diagnostic Radiology, Glostrup Hospital, Institute of Hygiene and Institute of Pathology, University of Copenhagen, DK-2600 Glostrup

Table 1. Number of particles allowed in 1 ml parenteral solution

	> 2 μm	> 5 μm	> 10 μm	> 25 μm
British Pharmacopeia 1973	1000	100		
United States Pharma-copeia XIX, 1975			50	5
Aircraft Industries [a]		35		

[a] Information taken from the regulation NAV-AIR-10-1A-17

intravenous infusions and found granulomas caused by the impurities. However, the clinical consequences of *intravenous* injection of manufacturing impurities from angiographic solutions and equipment are so negligible that they are not discussed here.

Several case reports deal with the risks and potential hazards of embolism during *arteriography* (*Brekkan* et al. 1975; *Chason* et al. 1963; *Hessel* et al. 1981; *Mani* and *Eisenberg* 1978 a, b; *Mani* et al. 1978; *Nehen* et al. 1978; *Olivecrona* 1977; *Schlossman* 1972; *Sigstedt* and *Lunderquist* 1978; *Silbermann* et al. 1960; *Zatz* and *Ianone* 1966). However, fundamental analysis of the inherent or endogenous particles in angiographic equipment such as solutions, catheters and guide-wires was only recently reported by *Winding* (1977, 1980; *Winding* and *Holma* 1976).

It is difficult indeed to understand that the most advanced documents of pharmaceutical legislation, the pharmacopoeias, are only slightly aware of these particulate impurities. For example, the *European Pharmacopoeia* of 1979 requires no more than: 'Solutions for injection, examined under suitable conditions of visibility, are clear and practically free from particles'. It is even more interesting that the *United States Pharmacopeia* (*Rockville* 1979) and the *British Pharmacopoeia* (1973) have much more liberal conditions regarding the particulate contamination of parenteral solutions than the standards required for hydraulic fluids in the American aircraft industry (Table 1).

Until recently investigations about the role of intra-arterial injection of manufacturing impurities were not available. Therefore, *Winding* and his colleagues investigated the biological significance of such particles in angiography of experimental animals (*Winding* et al. 1980). They closed the circle which began with in vitro studies of endogenous particulate contamination of ampoules, vials, catheters and guide-wires by finding identical particulate substances in thrombosed arteries of the rabbit kidneys investigated. Furthermore, using the intrinsic particles in contrast media as damaging agents the same team also studied the history of thrombo-embolism in the rabbit kidney, thus increasing knowledge about both the acute and chronic response of renal tissue to ischaemic damage (*Faarup* et al., in print).

In the following sections, information will be given about the different methods used for elucidation of the complex problems of finding, counting and determining foreign bodies in angiographic solutions and equipment (*Winding* 1977, 1980; *Winding* and *Holma* 1976). Subsequently an experimental model for assessment of the damage caused by these particles will be described (*Winding* et al. 1980) and finally the sequelae of lesions due to intra-arterial injection of the particulate impurities in the rabbit kidney will be documented (*Faarup* et al., to be published).

2 Materials and Methods

2.1 In Vitro

2.1.1 Solutions

Ten ampoules and ten vials of i.v. contrast media of all brands commercially available in Europe and normal saline from two manufacturers were investigated on a laminar air-flow bench under clean-room conditions ensuring extreme environmental purity. A Coulter counter was used to screen for particles according to size (>5 μm). *Winding* and *Holma* (1976) developed a specially designed cannula supplied with a plane membrane filter (Nuclepore) to collect particles exceeding 0.2 μm. This filter allowed direct transfer of the particles collected to a scanning electron microscope (SEM), which was directly connected to equipment for energy dispersive X-ray analysis (EDAX).

Thus the methods used allowed quantitation, shape analysis and substance determination of the particulate impurities in flushing solutions and contrast media.

2.1.2 Catheters and Guide-wires

Three brands of angiographic catheters of polyurethane and polyethylene and one brand of round-coil stainless steel guide-wire were investigated. The catheters were French no. 7 size with a length of 100 cm. The guide-wires were 120 cm long and 0.97 mm in diameter.

For quantitation of particles released, the catheters were flushed with 200-ml membrane-filtered, redistilled water. Particles were collected on plane membrane filters and then the guide-wire was inserted and withdrawn, followed by a second flushing with 20 ml filtered water. The particles released were collected as described above. After longitudinal cutting the internal surfaces of the catheters were studied under the light microscope and SEM. Randomly chosen single particles were analysed by means of EDAX for elements within the atomic numbers 9–93. Furthermore, ten randomly chosen specimens of 8 mm length from each catheter and guide-wire were investigated under the SEM.

In this experiment the collection of particles was also carried out on a laminar air-flow bench under clean-room conditions.

2.2 In Vivo

2.2.1 Quantitation of Lesions

Thirty-two male white Danish rabbits (average weight 2500 g) underwent transfemoral selective left renal arteriography under intravenous sodium pentobarbital

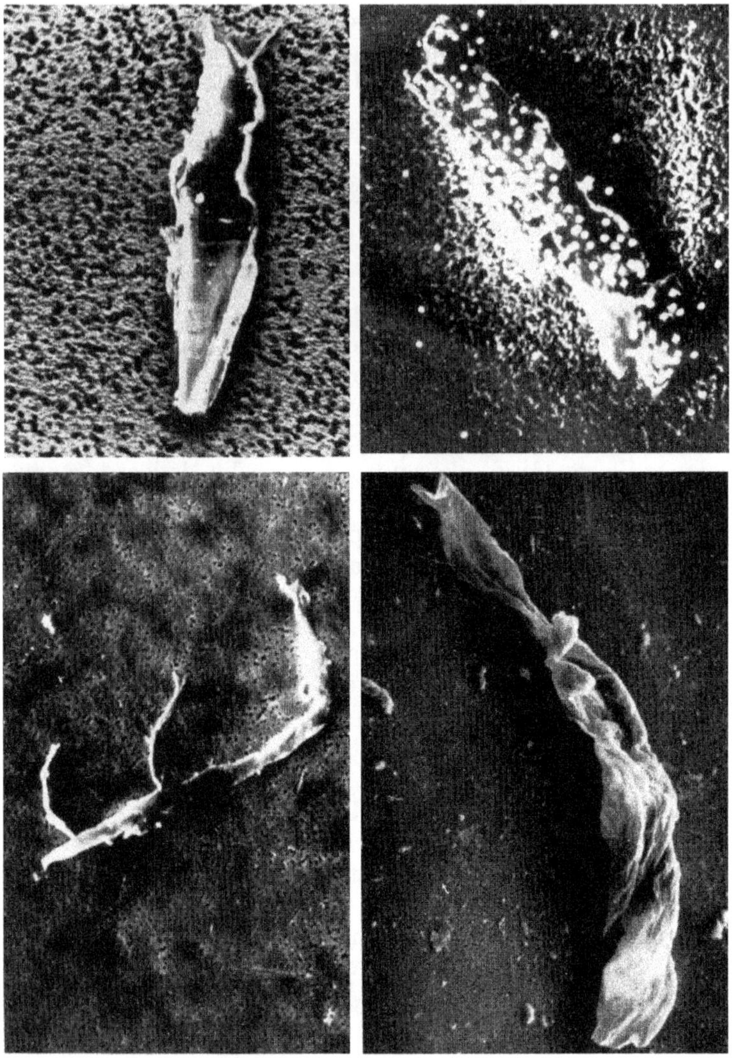

a b c d

Fig. 1 a–d. SEM images of particles found in contrast media at in vitro investigation. **a** glass 6 μm length; **b** metal particle photographed during EDAX procedure. Note the X-ray quanta; **c** organic fibre 11 μm length; **d** organic material, length 14 μm

anaesthesia according to *Adams* et al. (1965). Prior to the procedure the area was shaved, washed and the exposed artery was isolated. New catheters and guide-wires cleaned ultrasonically were used for each procedure. Before and during angiography the catheters were flushed with normal saline filtered through a 0.2-μm-pore-size membrane filter. Five different brands of water-soluble contrast media in glass ampoules were selected at random. Firstly angiography using 0.7–0.9 ml filtered (0.2-μm pore size) contrast medium was performed; immediately afterwards a further injection was given with an identical amount of contrast medium taken from the bottom of a 20-ml ampoule which had been previously centrifuged to concentrate the particles. After this angiography, the catheter was removed and the wound sutured. The urine from the animals was collected for 24 h and examined for blood. A repeat angiography was made with filtered contrast medium 3 days later in six rabbits, 14 days later in six and 21 days later in 11. A control group of nine rabbits underwent the same treatment using only filtered contrast medium.

Immediately after the repeat angiography both kidneys were removed for further investigation as follows: (a) macroscopic inspection and photography; (b) in seven kidneys microangiography, according to *Clark* et al. (1977); (c) microdisection of thrombi and foreign bodies guided by in vivo angiography and microangiography; (d) serial histological examination of tissues taken from both renal poles, from the central region and all affected areas; and (e) SEM and EDAX analysis of the particles isolated.

2.2.2 Sequelae

In 22 male white Danish rabbits transfemoral selective left renal angiography was performed under the same conditions as described for the previous experiment. One injection was given of 0.8 ml non-filtered contrast medium from the bottom of a 20-ml ampoule which had been previously centrifuged.

Three days after angiography the kidneys were carefully exposed at laparotomy and photographed from a standard distance. The diameter of affected areas found on the surface of the kidneys was measured. The wounds were sutured and the animals returned to routine conditions. Three weeks later at a second laparotomy the kidneys were exposed again, photographed from the standard distance and the diameter of surface damage measured.

All kidneys, including the contralateral kidneys, were then removed, fixed in 4% formalin buffer and examined histologically. Tissue was taken from the damaged areas seen both 3 days and 3 weeks after the angiographic procedure. All kidneys (including the contralaterals) were examined histologically as described previously. In four left kidneys microangiography was also performed.

3 Results

3.1 In Vitro

3.1.1 Solutions

Table 2 shows the results for normal saline used to flush angiographic catheters. Table 3 gives the quantities of foreign bodies in contrast media as determined by the Coulter counter. In Table 4 the results obtained by SEM are shown. Figure 1 shows examples of foreign bodies in contrast media as demonstrated by SEM.

EDAX analysis disclosed elements such as silicon, iodine, chromium, cobalt, iron, manganese, aluminium, calcium, chlorine, sodium, potassium and zinc in the particles. In a large number of fibre-like particles it was not possible to identify the composition of the substances, since the EDAX analysis can only pick up atomic numbers 9–93 in the periodic system. These fibres were presumably of organic material (cotton, plastic etc.).

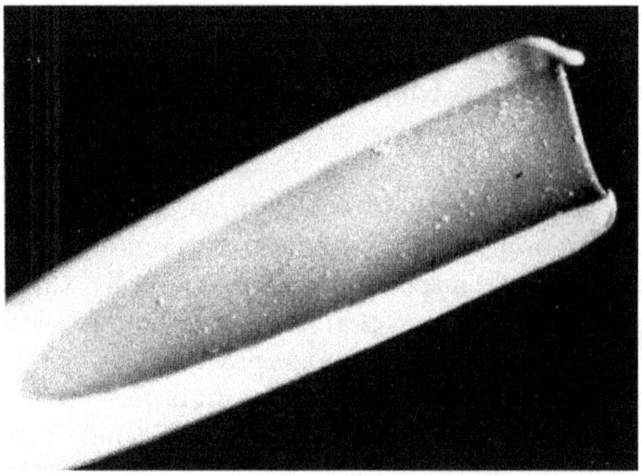

Fig. 2

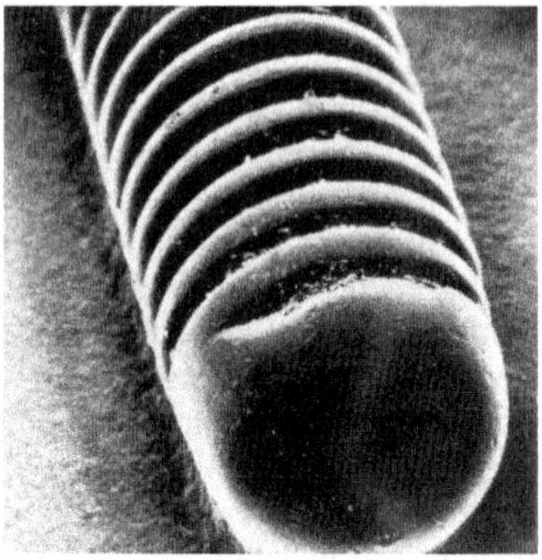

Fig. 3

Fig. 2. Unused sterile catheter tip cut longitudinally. Manufacturing debris is present in large amounts

Fig. 3. Tip of sterile unused guide-wire with high degree of contamination mostly trapped between the coils

Table 2. Number of particles on membrane filters after filtration of 1 l 0,9% normal saline from two manufacturers[a]

Manufacturer	< 0.5 µm	0.5–1 µm	1–5 µm	5–50 µm
A	212 500	151 785	25 000	3 571
B	137 750	81 250	32 142	8 928

[a] Mean values from 130 counts

Table 3. Number of particles in 1 ml contrast medium from five manufacturers as measured with Coulter counter[a]

Manufacturer		5–10 µm	10–30 µm	> 30 µm
A	Ampoules	258	79	1
	Vials	90	11	0
B	Ampoules	136	73	1
	Vials	107	25	1
C	Ampoules	301	171	3
	Vials	119	29	1
D	Ampoules	337	88	1
	Vials	36	6	1
E	Ampoules	394	124	1
	Vials	–	–	–

[a] Mean values of 50 measurements/brand

3.1.2 Catheters and Guide-wires

The surface characteristics and contamination of the catheters and guide-wires are shown in Figs. 2 and 3. Table 5 gives the levels of particles released from the unused catheters and Table 6 the levels of particles released from the catheters after one insertion of guide-wire.

3.2 In Vivo

3.2.1 Quantitation of Lesions

Radiologically and histopathologically detected lesions are listed in Table 7.

Of the 32 animals investigated 20 had postangiographic haematuria. In 16 kidneys arterial occlusions were found during in vivo angiography, and in four arteriovenous fistulae were also established (Fig. 4). Microangiography on five kidneys showed arterial obstructions, in two combined with bridging collaterals (Fig. 5). Microdissection disclosed the presence of thrombus-containing particles in 11 kidneys (Fig. 6). Furthermore, several infarctions of varying diameters were seen in all rabbits belonging to the groups killed 3 or 14 days after the initial angiography. However, in 4 of the 11 animals killed 21 days after the initial angiography no macroscopic lesions could be detected. In the control series more than half of the rabbit kidneys were free from morphological changes.

During serial histopathological investigation several small infarctions and ischaemic atrophic changes were found. Using polarising light microscopy hundreds of very small crystal-like particles were identified on the slides, some in thrombi, others in recanalized arterioles and capillaries (Fig. 7). In the contralateral right kidneys no pathological changes were found.

In the particles analyzed by SEM and EDAX silicon, phosphorus, iron and organic substances were found, similar in quality, distribution and pattern to those of the foreign bodies studied in vitro.

Table 4. Number of particles in 1 ml contrast medium from five manufacturers as measured with a scanning electron microscope

Manufacturer		5–10 μm	10–30 μm	> 30 μm
A	Ampoules	320	120	13
	Vials	61	45	5
B	Ampoules	310	125	8
	Vials	323	46	5
C	Ampoules	302	131	8
	Vials	369	183	3
D	Ampoules	370	322	13
	Vials	138	47	4
E	Ampoules	450	320	9
	Vials	–	–	–

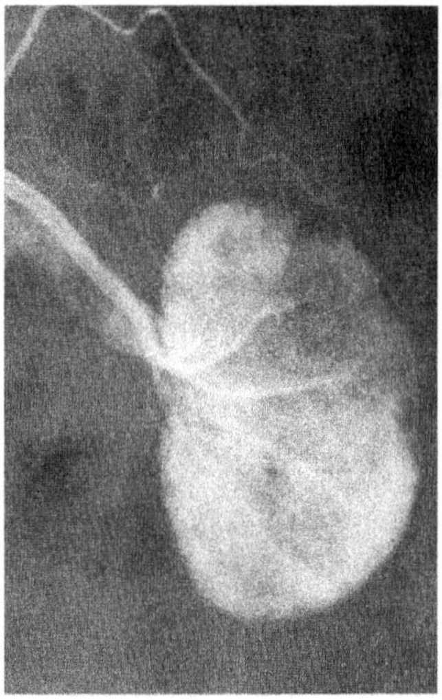

Fig. 4

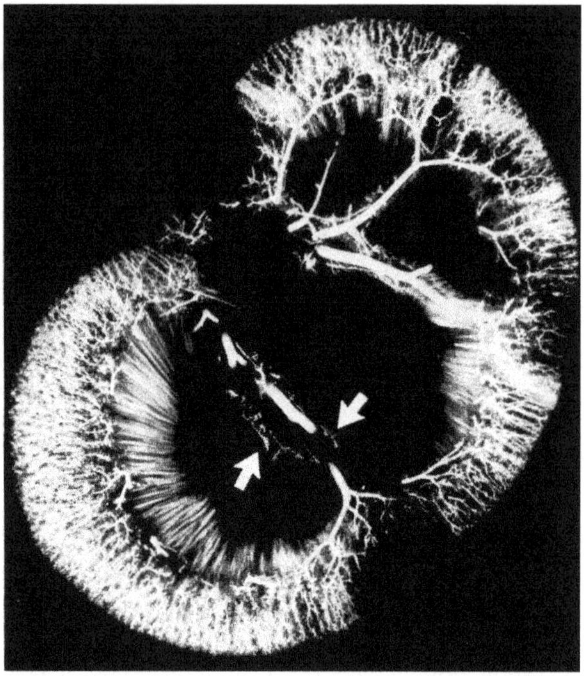

Fig. 5

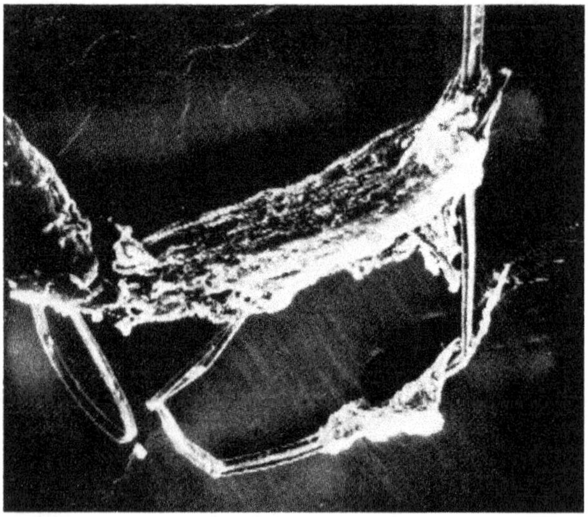

Fig. 6

Fig. 4. In vivo selective renal angiogram showing at least three cortical infarctions and arterio-venous fistula on the film exposed 1 s after injection

Fig. 5. Microangiography shows obstruction of a large artery and infarction of the area of supply. Note development of bridging collaterals (*arrows*)

Fig. 6. SEM image of thrombus removed from an arcuate artery containing a fibre-like particle

Fig. 7. a Microscopic image of an arteriole containing foreign bodies at the site of its division (*arrows*). A large particle (*double arrow*) is partially located in the media of the vascular wall. Recanalization changes are also present (*open arrow*). **b** Linear artefact formed during the histological preparation caused by removal of a crystalline foreign body from a glomerulus. *Insert,* the remaining part of the particle is still present in the neighbouring slide (*arrow*) ►

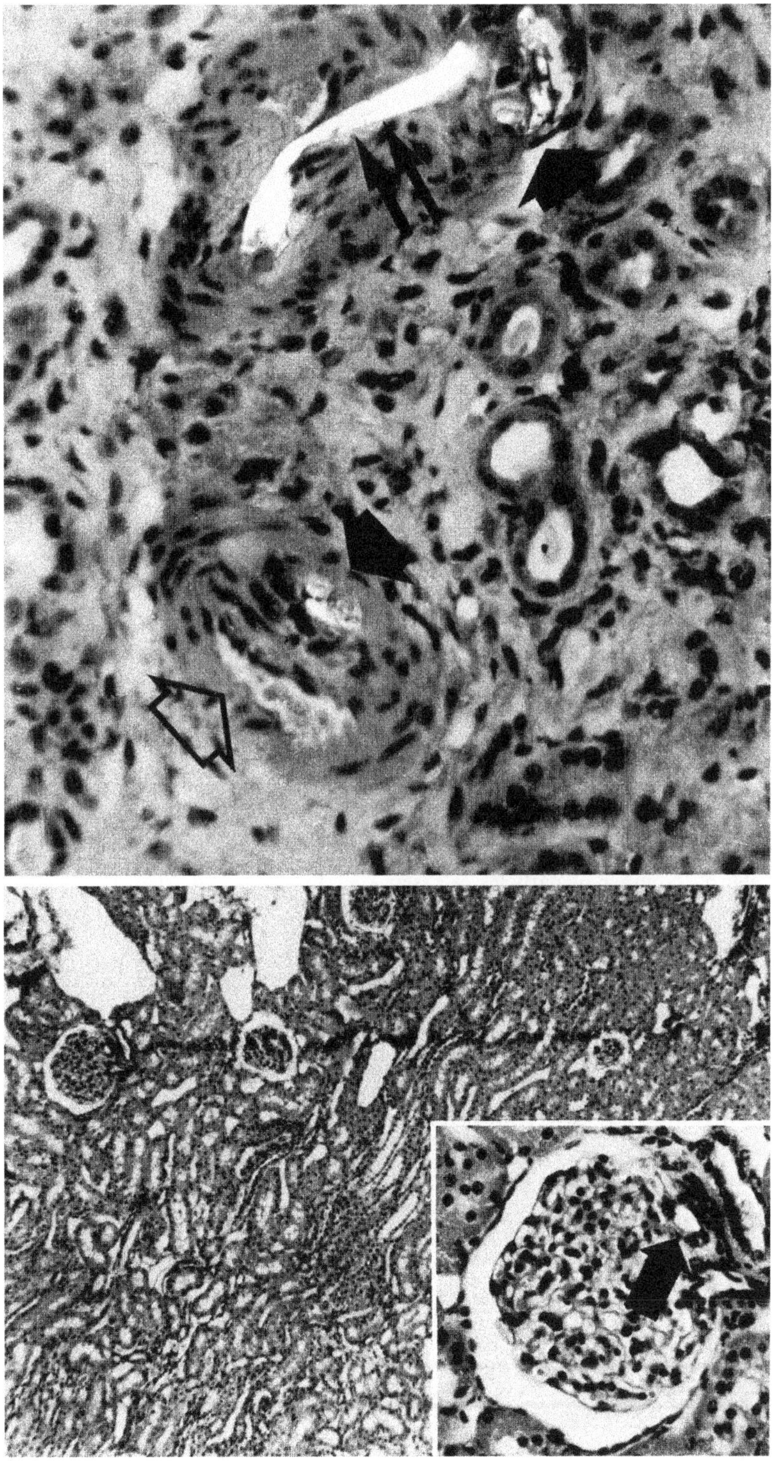

a

b

Fig. 7 a, b

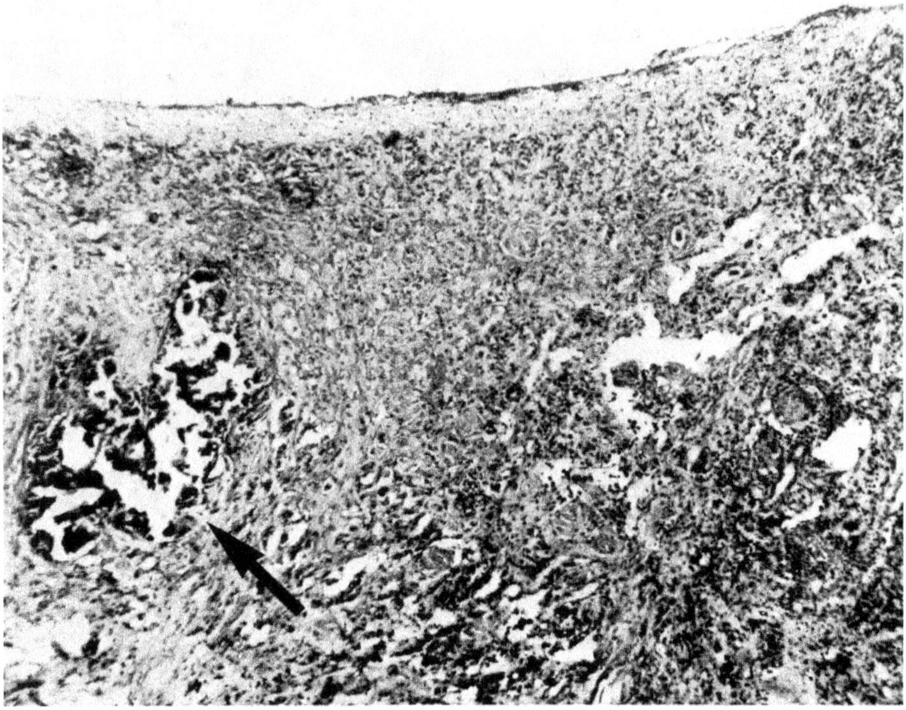

Fig. 8. Microscopy of typical old renal infarction more than 5 mm in diameter in which the parenchyma is replaced by fibrous tissue containing calcium deposits (*arrow*)

Table 5. Number of particles released after flushing with 20 ml filtered water from 100-cm angiographic catheters

Manufacturer		1–5 μm	5–10 μm	> 10 μm
A	Green	89 000	1000	500
B	Blue	42 000	500	500
C	Yellow	37 000	1500	1000

Table 6. Number of particles released from 100-cm angiographic catheters after one guide-wire insertion followed by flushing with 20 ml filtered water

Manufacturer [a]		1–5 μm	5–10 μm	> 10 μm
A	Green	450 000	7000	6000
B	Blue	220 000	8000	1000
C	Yellow	200 000	6000	3000

[a] Same brands as in Table 5

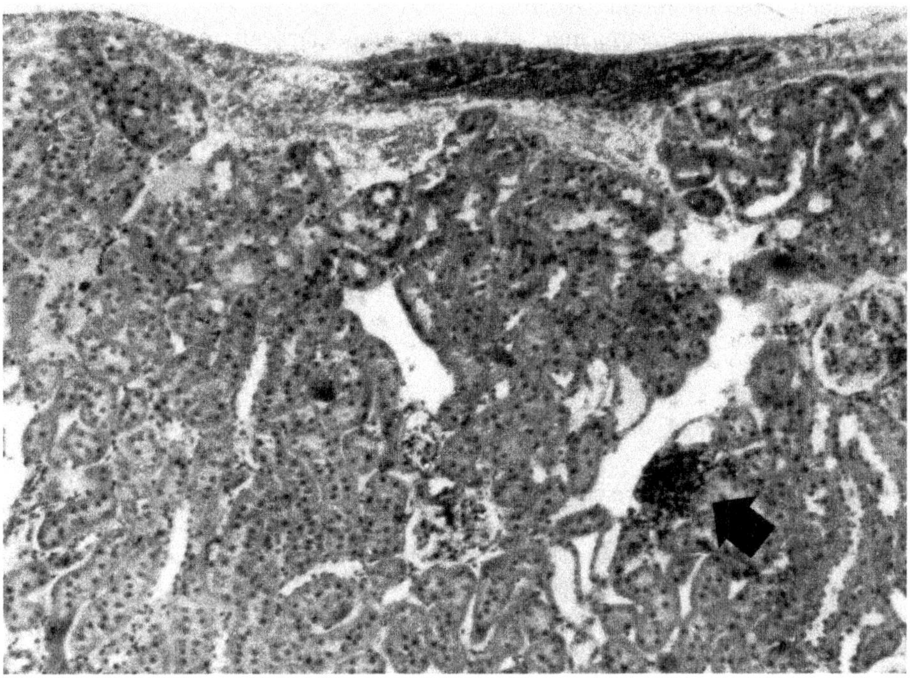

Fig. 9. Local tissue change 3 weeks after angiography in an area macroscopically less than 5 mm in diameter at first observation. Microscopy shows slight focal mononuclear infiltration (*arrow*), dilated vessels and minimal depression of the surface involved. Otherwise the parenchyma shows no significant pathological change

Table 7. Radiologically and histopathologically detected lesions in 32 rabbit kidneys

Groups		No. of rabbits	Lesions detected		Total	
			X-ray	Histology	No.	%
I	(3 days)	6	5	6	6	100
II	(14 days)	6	4	6	6	100
III	(21 days)	11	4	6	6	64
IV	(control)	9	3	4	4	45

3.2.2 Sequelae

In 19 of the 22 left kidneys a total of 21 surface changes were found 3 days after angiography; 19 were typical anaemic infarctions; while two appeared only as slightly pale, yet well-demarcated surface abnormalities. The changes varied in size from 2 mm diameter to involvement of more than the half the kidney.

Three weeks later the ten surface changes smaller than 5 mm in diameter disappeared. The 11 changes of more than 5 mm diameter showed typical signs of old, healed renal infarctions. Microscopy also showed several differences between the sequelae of the large and small infarctions. In the large infarctions hyalinisation of glomeruli, severe tubular atrophy, fibrosis and tissue shrinkage documented the known pattern of healed infarction (Fig. 8). In the small infarctions only borderline changes were present such as glomerular micro-aneurysm, localised tubular atrophy and slight interstitial fibrosis with occasional mononuclear infiltration (Fig. 9). However, in both groups of healed damage in the feeding arteries, foreign bodies, thrombi and recanalizations were found. Thus there were no significant differences in the aetiology of the fibrous healed infarctions and the functionally healed ones. Nevertheless, it was clearly demonstrated that minor ischaemic damage in the rabbit renal parenchyma has the ability to return to a more or less normal state.

4 Discussion and Conclusions

Several works deal with the chemistry, physiology and immunology of intravascular solutions and contrast media and there are further works describing the iatrogenic hazards of the angiographic procedure (*Adams* et al. 1969; *Hessel* et al. 1981; *Jacobson* and *Schlossman* 1969; *Mani* and *Eisenberger* 1978 a, b; *Mani* et al. 1978; *Olivecrona* 1977; *Schlossman* 1972; *Sigstedt* and *Lunderquist* 1978). Research has been carried out on the biological significance of artificially introduced microspheres into the vascular bed and the thrombogenicity of catheters (*Anderson* et al. 1974; *Axelsson* et al. 1977; *Bair* and *Petersen* 1979; *Bourossa* et al. 1976; *Casarella* 1977; *Forbes* and *Prentice* 1978; *Jacobson* and *Schlossman* 1969; *Rosenbusch* et al. 1977; *Schlossman* 1972; *Winding* 1981).

Damage caused by intrinsic particulate contamination of parenteral solutions and angiographic equipment was only previously described in the literature in case reports (*Adams* et al. 1965; *Chason* et al. 1963; *Nehen* et al. 1978; *Silbermann* et al. 1960; *Zatz* and *Lanone* 1966).

A systematic analysis of the contamination with intrinsic sterile particles of commercially available solutions and angiographic equipment and the biological significance of this contamination has been attempted in the investigations described here. The results of *Winding* and his co-workers also assess the complex problem of standards of hygiene in equipment used in the angiographic procedure (*Winding* 1977, 1980, 1981; *Winding* and *Holma* 1976; *Winding* et al. 1980).

Over the years tons of contrast media, saline and other drugs have been flushed through the human arterial tree using kilometres of catheters and guide-wires. Although angiographic damage in man is usually registered in the hospital charts we cannot know with confidence how much of this is related to the manufacturing impurities of the equipment used. However, occasional reports, insurance and court cases indicate that such types of damage to the human body do occur.

Therefore, further investigation of the large number of clinical cases should be made. However, already at this point some conclusions can be drawn after discussion of the following questions:

1. Can the damage to the rabbit kidney examined in these experiments provide direct conclusions about the reactions of human tissue?

2 Can tissue damage caused by the physical properties of parenteral solutions and angiographic equipment be avoided or at least decreased?

1. The size of the rabbit inhibits the use of equivalent contrast doses to those used in man. Therefore, the particulate content of 20 ml contrast medium – being comparable with the doses used in human selective renal angiography – was concentrated in a smaller volume. Since large amounts of identical particles were found in the renal arteries, there is no doubt that the damage was caused by foreign body emboli. – Why is similar damage following human selective renal angiography not seen to the same extent? The answer is difficult and only poorly documented. However, postangiographic haematuria is well known to every radiologist and still remains unexplained (*Lindholm* 1979). At least in some cases such transitional haematuria could be explained by small emboli. Furthermore, major damage to the rabbit kidney was caused by emboli in the main renal artery or in its primary branches, which are comparable in size to the human interlobar and arcuate arteries, respectively. In the much larger volume of the human body and kidney the amount of superimposed substance makes it difficult to detect in the films small lesions in a few arcuate arteries and impossible in the interlobular arteries. Even in small rabbits post-mortem microangiography of thin slices of kidneys and a specific microscopic technique were necessary in the majority of our investigations in order to find the thrombi and the foreign bodies.

One of the most interesting results of the experiments concerned the regenerative ability of the rabbit kidney parenchyma. Although there is no clear statement about the similarity of the rabbit and the human kidney it can be assumed that similar healing tendencies also exist in the human kidney. In the rabbit kidneys small infarct-like changes after angiography disappeared at least to the extent that only microscopy could reveal small atrophic changes in the nephrons involved, indicating recovery to a functioning state. Recanalisation of vessels and development of collaterals could be demonstrated in many cases already within 1 week after establishment of thrombus. Since the rabbit kidney possesses end-arteries like the human kidney, there is good reason to assume that the observations in the rabbit kidney can be of a more general value, possibly also applying to man. Thus the conclusions of the material documented here are twofold. Yes, the manufacturing impurities can cause damage with severe sequelae including loss of functioning tissue. On the other hand, the vast majority of damage is caused by very small particles (Tables 2–6), probably followed by reversible changes. Thus careful handling of angiography in respect to both indication and technique during the procedure should be expected.

2. Is it possible to avoid the damage caused by the manufacturing impurities of solutions, catheters and guidewires? – Despite remarkable attention to, and progress in, production only slight improvements have been achieved in the manufacturing process. However, by keeping to some basic rules during the angiographic procedure the number of large particles introduced into the arteries can be decreased. Vials should be opened by removing the cap and not by penetrating the membrane, since the needle usually pushes large rubber particles into the solution. Ampoules contain a vacuum; therefore, when they are opened large glass particles will escape into the solution. After a short time these sink to the bottom. They can

be avoided if the end of the suction needle is kept above the bottom of the ampoule and approximately 3 mm of the bottom layer is not used. Furthermore, the solutions should be filtered as far as possible in the angiographic procedure. In our experience, effective filtration at injection with power syringes during human angiography cannot be carried out without influencing the flow. However, it is possible to fill the syringe through a filter (5-μm pore size), although it is a demanding and slow process.

For catheters and guide-wires it is necessary that the guide-wire be moved in and out a few times inside the dry catheter followed by high pressure flushing of the catheter several times. By this manipulation loose debris from the catheter lumen is removed. The guide-wire has to be rinsed in large amounts of water and not dried with a gauze pad. Furthermore, bending the catheter when it is moved over the guide-wire should be avoided. The friction of the hard metal against the soft plastic increases considerably when bent, and long plastic shavings (maximum 3.8 cm, in our experience) can be scraped from the wall of the catheter and released into the artery.

Finally, great attention should be paid to increasing the strictness of indications for *diagnostic* angiography. Whenever possible non-invasive methods should be used for such purposes, while angiography should be increasingly reserved for *therapeutic* purposes. The material we present here is based on experimental research; however, its significance for human patients is more or less founded on hypothesis. The authors hope to stimulate further research into daily routine clinical work to find results of sufficient significance for appropriate placement of angiography in the increasing armoury of diagnostic imaging.

References

Adams DF, Olin TB, Kosek J (1965) Cotton fiber embolization during angiography. A clinical and experimental study. Radiology 84:678–681

Anderson JH, Gianturco C, Wallace S, Dodd GD (1974) A scanning electron microscopic study of angiographic catheters and guide-wires. Radiology 111:567–571

Axelsson H, Schonebeck J, Winblad B (1977) Surface structure of unused and used catheters. Scand J Urol Nephrol 11:283–287

Bair JN, Petersen RV (1979) Surface characteristics of plastic intravenous catheters. Am J Hosp Pharm 36:1701–1711

Bourossa MG, Cantin M, Sandborn EB, Pederson E (1976) Scanning electron microscopy of surface irregularities and thrombogenesis of polyurethane and polypropylene coronary catheters. Circulation 53:992–996

Brekkan A, Lexow PE, Woxholt G (1975) Glass fragment and other particles contaminating contrast media. Acta Radiol [Diagn] (Stockh) 16:600–608

British Pharmacopoeia (1973) Pharmaceutical Press, London

Casarella WJ (1977) Guide wire thrombogenicity measured by fibrinopeptide A radioimmunoassay. Am J Roentgenol 128:363–368

Chason JL, Landers JW, Swanson RE (1963) Cotton fiber embolism. A frequent complication of cerebral angiography. Neurology 13:558–560

Clark RL, Mandel SR, Webster WP (1977) Microvascular changes in canine renal allograft rejection: A correlative microangiographic and histologic study. Invest Radiol 12:62–73

European Pharmacopoeia (1979) Counsil of Europe. Maisonneuve SA, Paris

Faarup P, Winding O, Pilapil A, Grønvall J, Hegedüs V (in print) Reversible changes in small infarcts of the rabbit kidney. Scand J Urol Nephrol

Forbes CD, Prentice CRM (1978) Thrombus formation and artificial surface. Br Med Bull 34:201–207

Garvan JM, Gunnar BW (1963) Intravenous fluids: A solution containing such particles must not be used. Med J Aust 2:140–146

Garvan JM, Gunnar BW (1964) The harmful effects of particles in intravenous fluids. Med J Aust 2:1–6

Hessel SI, Adams DF, Abrams MD (1981) Complications of Angiography. Radiology 138: 273–281

Idbohrn H, Berg N (1954) On the tolerance of the rabbit's kidney to contrast media in renal angiography. A roentgenologic and histologic investigation. Acta Radiol [Diagn] (Stockh) 42:121–140

Jacobson B (1969) Platelet adhesion and aggregation following contact between blood and vascular catheters in vitro. Scand J Haemat 6:216–220

Jacobson B, Schlossman D (1969) Thromboembolism of leg following percutaneous catheterization of femoral artery for angiography. Acta Radiol [Diagn] (Stockh) 8:109–118

Mani RL, Eisenberg RL (1978a) Complications of catheter cerebral arteriography: Analysis of 5000 procedures. II: Relation of complication rates to clinical and arteriographic diagnoses. AJR 131:867–869

Mani RL, Eisenberg RL (1978b) Complications of catheter cerebral arteriography: Analysis of 5000 procedures. III: Assessment of arteries injected, contrast medium used, duration of procedure, and age of patient. AJR 131:871–874

Mani RL, Eisenberg RL, McDonald EJ, Pollock JA, Mani JR (1978) Complications on catheter cerebral arteriography: Analysis of 5000 procedures. I: Criteria and incidence. AJR 131:861–865

Nehen AM, Damgaard-Jensen L, Hansen PE (1978) Foreign body embolism of retinal arteries as a complication of carotid angiography. Neuroradiology 15:82–85

Olivecrona H (1977) Complications of cerebral angiography. Neuroradiology 14:175–181

Panum PL (1862) Untersuchungen über den plötzlichen Tod durch Embolie mittels der durch die selbe gesetzten Unterbrechung des Blutstromes. Arch Pathol Anat 25:310–338

Rockville (1979) The United States Pharmacopoeia. US Pharmacopoeial convention 1975. 19th Revision. 5th supplement

Rosenbusch G, Vincent J, van Douveren W, Penn Wm, Kuypers PJF, Arts THM (1977) Auslösung von intrarenal lokalisierten renorenalen Kollateralen beim Hund. Bemerkungen zum Endarteriencharakter der Nierenarterie. Fortschr Geb Roentgenstr Nuklearmed 126:407–417

Schlossman D (1972) Thrombogenicity of vascular catheters. Thesis. Gothenburg, Sweden

Sigstedt B, Lunderquist A (1978) Complications of angiographic examinations. AJR 130: 455–460

Silbermann J, Gravioto H, Feigim I (1960) Foreign body emboli following cerebral angiography. Arch Neurol 119–125

Thomas WH, Lee YK (1974) Particles in intravenous solutions, a review. N Z Med J 80: 170–178

Virchow R (1856) Gesammelte Abhandlungen zur Wissenschaftlichen Medicin. Meidinger

Williams A, Barnett MI (1973) Particulate contamination in intravenous fluids, administration sets and cannulae. Pharm J 211:190–204

Winding O (1977) Foreign bodies in contrast media for angiography. Am J Hosp Pharm 34:705–708

Winding O (1980) Intrinsic particles in angiographic contrast media. Radiology 134:317–320

Winding O (1981a) Particle release from angiographic utensils. Eur J Radiol 1:114–116

Winding O (1981b) Cerebral microembolization in rabbits following carotid injections of dextran microspheres. Neuroradiology 21:123–126

Winding O, Holma B (1976) Method for determination and element analysis of particulate contamination in injectable solutions. Am J Hosp Pharm 33:1154–1159

Winding O, Grønvall J, Faarup P, Hegedüs V (1980) Sequelae of intrinsic foreign-body contamination during selective renal angiography in rabbits. Radiology 134:321–326

Zatz LM, Ianone AM (1966) Cerebral emboli complicating cerebral angiography. Acta Radiol [Diagn] (Stockh) 5:621–630

Digital Radiography Using a Computed Tomography Instrument *

K.-H. Hübener [1]

1 Medizinisches Strahleninstitut, Universität Tübingen, Röntgenweg 11, D-7400 Tübingen

* With the kind support of the German Radiological Society (Deutsche Röntgengesellschaft), the German Research Community (Deutsche Forschungsgemeinschaft) and Siemens, A.G., Erlangen

1 Introduction

Attempts to utilize the techniques of digital processing in the field of diagnostic radiology were first made more than 20 years ago. At that time, efforts were made to digitize the information contained in the radiographic film, with the view – in addition to reducing the space requirement for filing purposes — of making possible a subsequent manipulation of the radiographic image. It was, however, recognized that the point-by-point scanning of the X-ray image required for the optical analog-digital conversion was unable to provide any information that was not already contained within the image. The point-by-point digital transformation, therefore, must always result in a loss of information.

The dream of obtaining digital radiographic images was stimulated by the tremendous progress in the field of electronic engineering over the last 2 decades that made it possible for the first time to utilize to the full the possibilities and advantages of digital in comparison with analog data processing modes. The fundamentals of a digitization of analog magnitudes are by no means the "invention" of computer engineering; rather, nature itself began to utilize the advantages of this technique at a very early stage of evolutionary development.

Sense perception and the transmission of stimuli employ this principle in all living creatures. Thus, for example, an acoustic signal received at the ear is first conducted along the external auditory meatus and then, after analog coupling (impedance matching), is conveyed across the tiny ossicles of the middle ear to the acoustic receptors of the inner ear. Here, the analog magnitude intensity of sound is frequency modulated in such a way that a strong (loud) signal (high signal amplitude) is transformed into a large number of uniform electrical impulses via electrochemical transmitter substances, while a quiet signal is converted into a series of lower frequency identical uniform signals. This type of analog-digital transformation is characteristic of the principle of digital processing (Fig. 1).

In the inner ear, further digital transformations take place, the perceived frequency spectrum being further decoded and processed, on the basis of a detailed frequency analysis (similar to a Fourier analysis).

This conversion of sensory stimuli into digitized uniform electrical signals, the action potentials, is met with in all the sense organs and throughout the stimulus-conducting system. This situation reflects the fact that a digital signal is far less susceptible to interference than an analog signal, that is, the information content of a stimulus, which is the actual "element" being transmitted, is more reliably preserved by this mode of signal processing than would be the case with simple analog processing. In nature, a uniform action potential of variable frequency can be transmitted across numerous nerves and synapses: at each synapse, the signal, weakened during transmission, again produces a uniform electrical pulse, the frequency and thus the carrier of the information, remaining uninfluenced.

These advantages of largely interference-free signal processing involving uniform pulses represent the basis for modern digital processing modalities. This latter combines the low susceptibility to interference with ease of data processing. The progress made in electronic data "perception", handling and reproduction are based on these advantages.

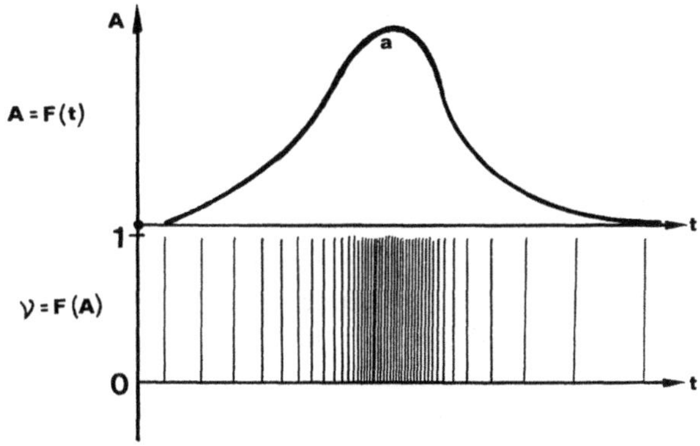

Fig. 1. The principle of analog digital conversion: a time-variable analog signal A = F(t) having the amplitude *a* is transformed into a proportional frequency ν of uniform impulses: ν = F(A)

The rapid development of electronics has also made it possible to rethink the question of their use in radiological engineering. Thus, from the considerations mentioned at the beginning of this article (the optical breakdown of an analog radiographic image), and the associated shortcomings, it could be concluded that a conversion of the analog X-ray signal following its passage through the body of the patient must be made at the beginning of the signal processing stage, in order to keep the ensuing loss of information to a minimum.

One possible way of achieving this objective is to be seen in the electronic processing of information made possible by an image intensifier fluoroscopic chain employing data recording facilities. This technology which, in comparison with X-ray film images, involves a reduction in the spatial and density resolution, is now employed in the technique of *"Digital Vascular Imaging"*, or *"Digital Fluoroscopy"*, which, today, is being employed only for the representation of the blood vessels with the aid of the subtraction technique (arteriography) following the transvenous administration of contrast medium.

The technique of digital radiography, which is being presented here, makes use of a computerized tomographic device (scanner) for the recording of X-ray beam attenuation employing a stationary imaging unit. In 1975, *Stein* proposed that such transmission profiles of the body should be obtained by employing a large single crystal having a length of 50 cm and an X-ray beam broken up, both spatially and temporally, into pulses by a rotating disc containing slits (collimator). Even the setup developed by *Stein* was able to demonstrate the decisive advantages of this procedure:

1. An extremely low radiation exposure of the patient (about 400 μR)
2. An almost complete lack of scattered radiation, and thus improved contrast

Practical experience with this setup was first described by *Curtis* in 1979. He used this digital "scanning unit" to carry out examinations in 18 polytraumatized patients, and was able to visualize all the major pathological changes that were decisive for the emergency treatment. For example, all fractures associated with dislocation (of the fragments) were demonstrated, and a case of pneumothorax reliably diagnosed.

1.1 Present-day Technology[1]

The digital radiographic setup employing a single crystal as a detector was not developed further. With the introduction of computerized tomographic scanners, in particular those of the third and fourth generations, the technical prerequisites for the production of digital radiographs with a similar setup have now been available since 1977/1978.

The CT scanners make use of a stationary gantry. The X-ray tube, located in a frontal or a lateral position and producing a fan-shaped beam, emits high-frequency pulsed X-rays. The attenuated X-radiation is detected by an array of detectors. By suitably collimating the X-ray beam, both at the tube and the detector side, it is ensured that only a very narrow X-ray beam having a width of 1–2 mm passes through the body of the patient. Furthermore, the geometrical arrangement is such that scattered radiation is virtually prevented from entering the detectors.

With the aid of this imaging setup (Fig. 2), a transversal transmission profile of a very narrow slice through the body can be imaged and stored. The transverse resolution within the body correlates with the size of the detectors. In the scanner discussed here, semiconductor detectors with coupled photodiodes having a width of 1.2 mm are employed. The imaging of *one* such transversal profile, however, does not permit any diagnostic interpretation to be made. In addition, measurements of the attenuation in the longitudinal direction of the body must also be made in order, on the basis of an electronic synthesis, to obtain a radiograph.

In practice, the patient is moved through the imaging unit at a speed of between 2.5 and 6 cm/s. During this procedure, the X-ray tube emits radiation in defined increments – generally of 1 mm. In this way, transversal attenuation profiles are obtained at 1 mm increments along the longitudinal axis of the patient's body.

The relatively large detectors for the longitudinal axis of the body (in the scanner discussed, the length of the detectors was 13.5 mm) make it necessary that only the differences of two contiguous transversal attenuation profiles 1 mm apart are utilized as the contribution of this thin slice through the body, to the attenuation of the X-ray beam. In this way, also for the longitudinal axis of the body, a digital grid can be obtained, which, at 1 mm, is suitable for the limits of spatial resolution of the transversal scanning direction (Fig. 3).

With the aid of the transmission profiles obtained in the transverse axis of the body, and the consecutive data for the X-ray attenuation obtained on moving the patient through the scanner, it is possible, on the basis of storage and further mathematical manipulations, to "put together" a digital radiograph. It is also possible to envisage imaging systems that function independently of a computerized tomographic unit, in which the appropriate data are obtained, by moving not the patient, but the imaging unit itself. Technically, it is also possible to construct imaging systems in which the patients do not have to be recumbent. Thus, an optimization of the technology for the production of digital radiographs makes numerous improvements appear feasible, which would not be possible in the case of data acquisition with a CT setup.

1 The technical details described were obtained by performing measurements on the Siemens CT scanner Somatom SF, the digital radiography produced by which are termed "Topogramms"

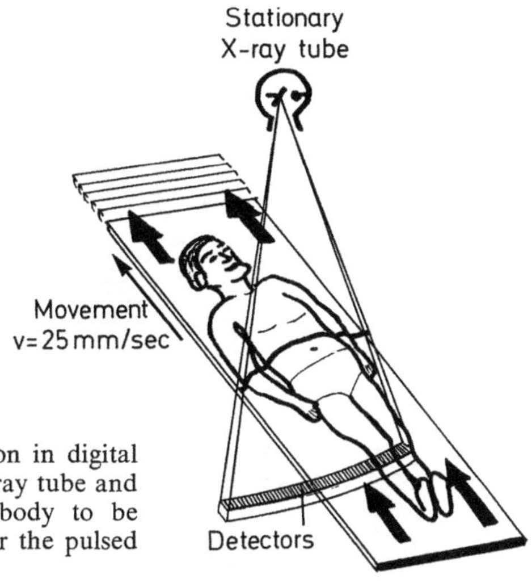

Fig. 2. Schematic drawing of image production in digital radiography using a CT scanner. With the X-ray tube and detector array stationary, the part of the body to be examined is moved at a constant speed under the pulsed X-ray fan beam

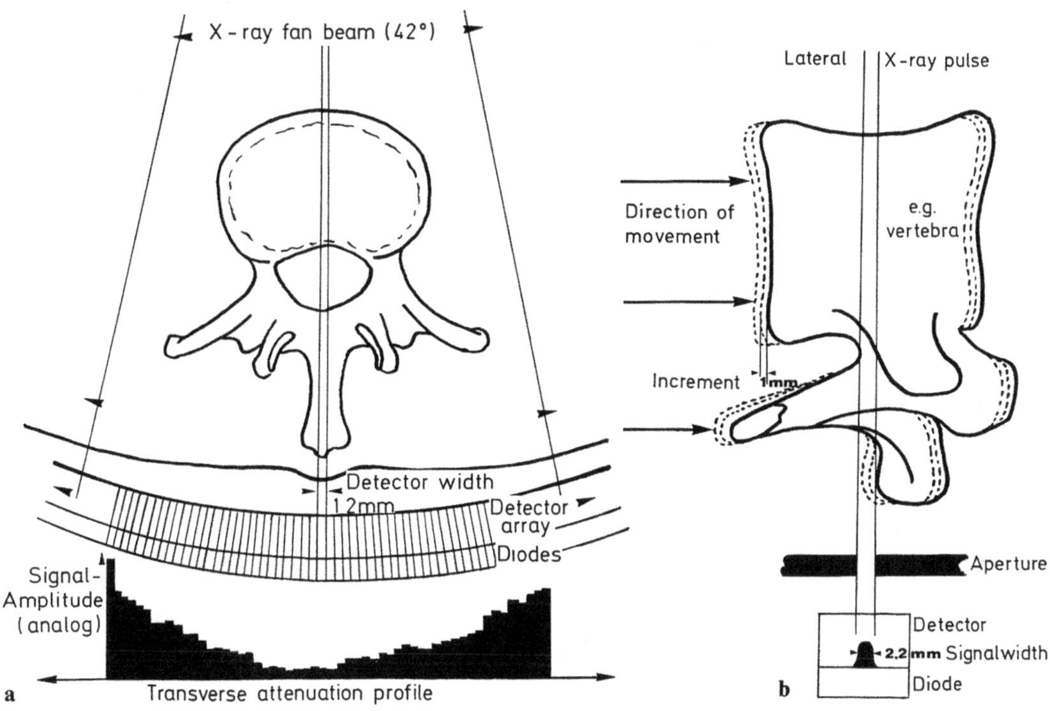

Fig. 3. a True-to-scale representation of the measured value recording (data collection) in the transversal section. Matching the attenuation of the object (for example, a vertebral body), a transversal attenuation profile is recorded and stored. **b** Analog representation in the longitudinal axis of the body. The movement of the patient is also represented schematically

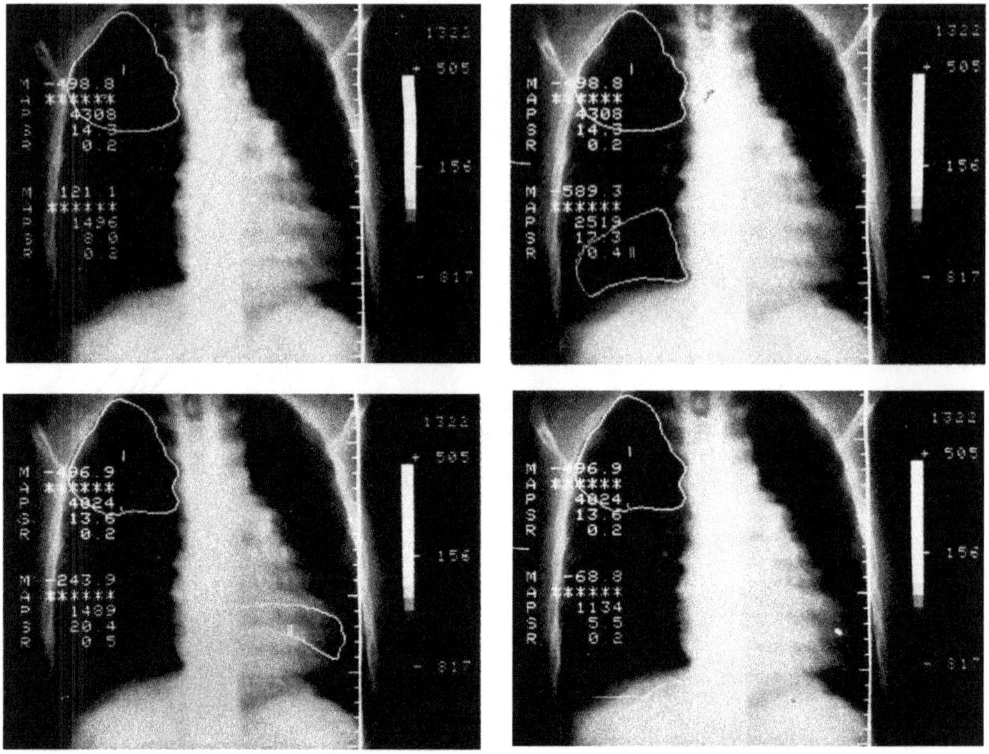

Fig. 4. Unfiltered radiographs which have been "put together" from the original transversal attenuation profiles. Also visualized are attenuation value measurements over various sections of the organs of the chest. The level marked *M* represents the mean attenuation value in the area indicated

With the exception of the attenuation profiles in the transversal and longitudinal axes of the body, the data can be used to produce a digital radiograph. With such a data matrix, which is not subjected to further processing, however, owing to the spectral dynamics of the detector array, a radiographic image that is difficult to interpret results (Fig. 4). Since the detectors permit a differentiation of the X-ray attenuation in about 20 000 steps, and these steps can be only very inadequately translated into the approximately 20 grey steps of a television monitor, it is generally necessary to "compress" the recorded data spectrum in such a way that the eye is presented with an evaluable radiograph that is normally compatible with the conventional X-ray image. The result of the necessary mathematical manipulations, however, a reduction in the information available on data acquisition, must be taken into consideration. Our experience shows, however, that, for the utilization of the advantages of this radiographic procedure, 500–1000 attenuation values (representing a reduction of the originally discriminated attenuation spectrum by the factor 1:20) suffice.

For certain medical problems, however, it is desirable that the entire dynamic spectrum of the data be available. Then, however, adjustment of the window

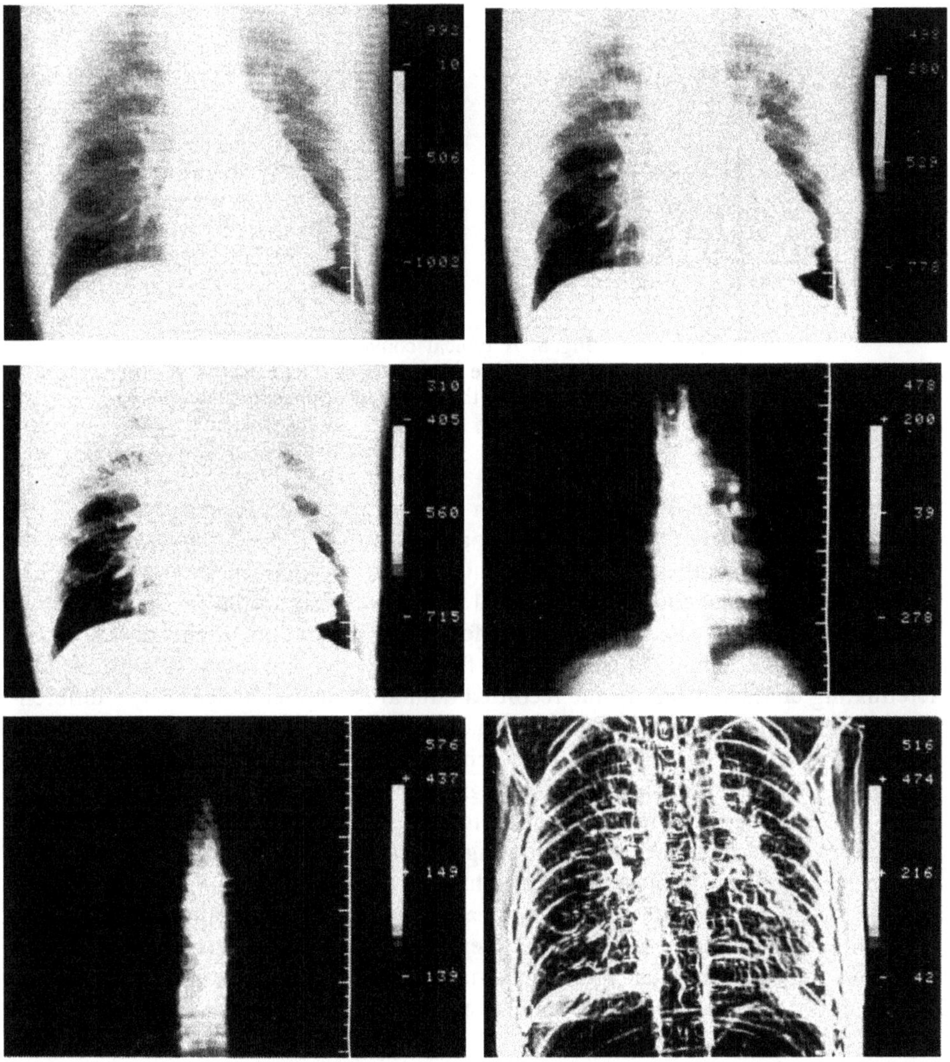

Fig. 5. Various window settings of the unfiltered digital radiographs show that to make full use of all the information, a considerable variation of the window setting and window width is necessary

position, and window width – analogous to computerized tomographic exposures – is necessary if all the available information is to be utilized fully (Fig. 5).

In the realization of easily interpretable digital radiographs, preference is given to pragmatic considerations. The reduction of data is carried out in such a manner that a radiograph similar to the well-known X-ray image is obtained. The original, so-called raw data, may be compressed in the process. A further possibility consists of a mathematical processing of the raw data. Here, for example, the original set of data can be convoluted with the aid of a mathematical function for each individual

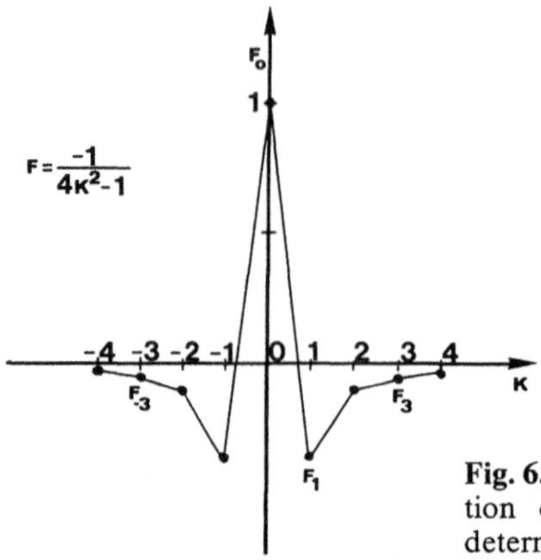

Fig. 6. A typical convolution function for the reconstruction of the radiographs. The factor *K* (filter kernel) determines the steepness of the density gradient

measured value. Today, this is a common way of proceeding, and the nature of the computation employed varies. Thus, for convolution, those functions that are employed in the "synthesis" (reproduction) of the computerized tomogram can also be used. In particular those mathematical algorithms that are useful for the filtered back projection can also be employed for the computation of the digital radiograph. These mathematical convolution functions have an almost exclusively differentiating character, that is, the recorded data are "edge-enhanced" by a differentiation of the measured data (Fig. 6). Thanks to the variability of the convolution functions, marked edge effects can be achieved, and these can lead to an easy-to-interpret pictorial impression in the radiograph.

A disadvantage of this differentiating image reconstruction, however, is the marked overshooting and undershooting effect at object structures of differing density (e.g. the transition between the lungs and the diaphragm, or between the wall of the thorax and air), which can lead to artefacts and "empty zones" within the radiograph. It has thus proved very expedient to mix the recorded sets of raw data and the mathematically filtered data sets. We generally employ a standard mixing ratio of these two components of 1 : 1. Other mixing ratios considerably modify the image impression (Fig. 7).

These mathematical manipulations of the data influence the integral attenuation figures considerably. In any case, since they represent summation values, they do not have the same degree of significance as in the transversal imaging of overlapping-free computerized tomograms. Since, both in the recording of transmission profiles and in the film image, the integral X-ray attenuation is summated in an unknown manner that depends upon the density and thickness of the patient's body, the attenuation figures measured in digital radiography can also be utilized to only a small degree. Increases or decreases in density can be "employed" usefully both visually and by using technical measuring means, only for a comparison of the two sides. In this connection, all the well-known measuring procedures (measuring points, areas, ROI) familiar in computerized tomography are available.

The data that "belong" to a digital radiograph can be suitably stored in the same way as that employed in computerized tomography. The data sets can be

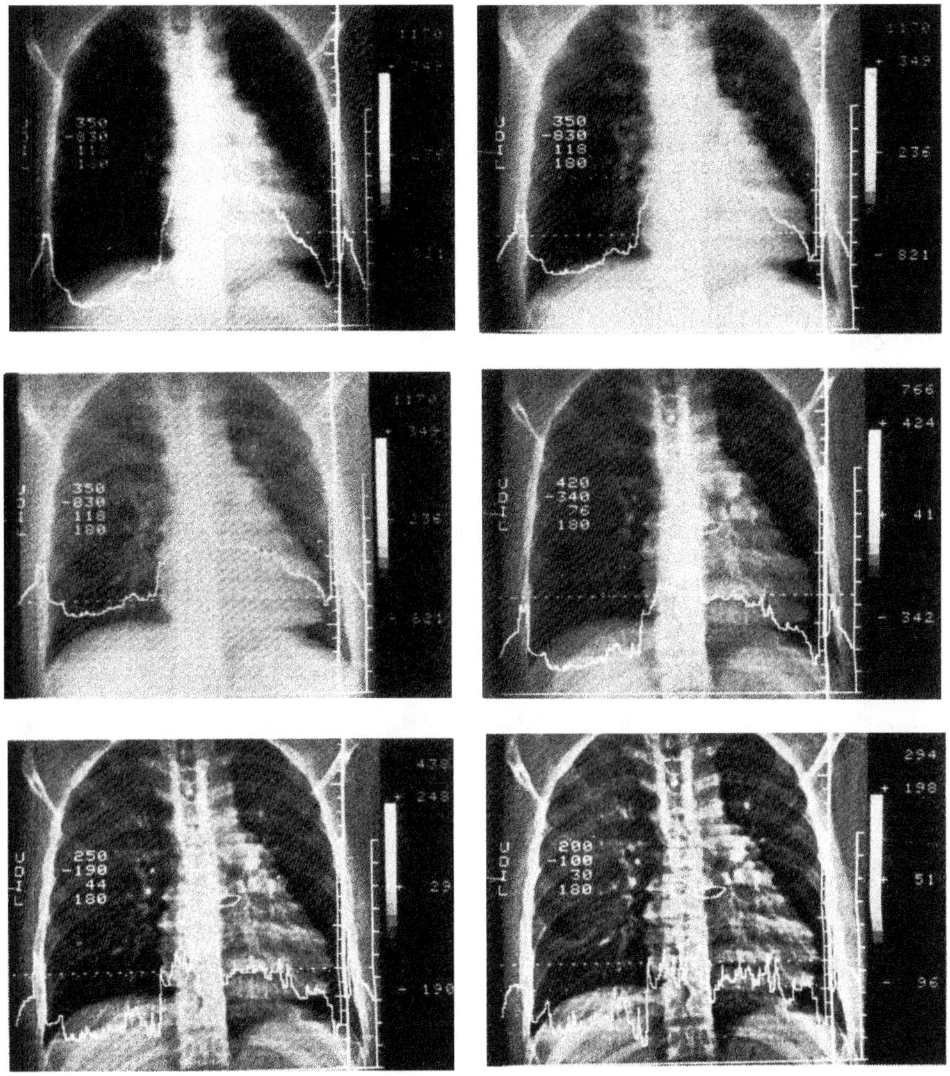

Fig. 7. The identical digital radiographic view with various mixing ratios, of unfiltered and convoluted measuring profiles. Overlapping by the attenuation value histogram obtained at the same level reveals that, by means of convolution and mixing, a reduction and shift in the absorption value scale result

stored on the conventional data carriers (floppy disk, magnetic disk or magnetic tape) and can be called up at any time. It can be envisaged that, as digital engineering spreads, transmission of these data to any point at which a television monitor can be installed will be also possible in the field of diagnostic radiology. Furthermore, long-distance transmission of the data contained in these radiographs, that is, transmission via radio or cable, will also present no problems.

2 Radiation Exposure, Spatial and Density Resolution, Errors and Artefacts

2.1 Dose Measurements

In the radiographic installation described by *Stein* (1975), in which a large single crystal (NaI crystal having a length of 54 cm and a diameter of 40 mm) an almost 100% absorption of the radiation was to be expected. The required number of quanta in the detector, and thus also the radiation exposure, attained a minimum of 2.5–3.5 μGy. The caesium iodide crystals used in the installation under investigation, each having a volume of $1.2 \times 13.5 \times 10\ mm^3$, permit a radiation utilization of about 77%.

In order to obtain an evaluable measuring signal in the detector – and in particular for the complete utilization of the measured value dynamics of 1:20000 – a minimum number of quanta are required in the detector to achieve the necessary signal-to-noise ratio.

For the desired dynamic range of 1:20000, about 10^7 quanta need to be registered. At an effective energy of 60 keV (125 kVp), this number of quanta represents an energy flow of 6×10^{11} eV. If a detector surface area of $0.12 \times 0.22\ cm^2$ is assumed, the energy flow density involved is $6 \times 10^{11}/0.0264\ eV/cm^2$.

At 60 keV, 1 R = 3000 erg/cm^2, so that the 10^7 quanta correspond to a dose of $D = \frac{0.6 \times 1.602}{0.264 \times 3000}\ R = 0.012\ R$. If the total detector surface area is assumed to be $1.35 \times 0.12\ cm^2 = 0.162\ cm^2$, an ion dose of R = 0.002 R = 2 mR, and an energy dose (1 R ≙ 1 rd) D = 2 mrd = 20 μGy, is obtained.

Dose measurements were carried out using condenser ionization chambers ("Kondiometer")[1] in an Alderson phantom in the chest and abdominal region. In order to make use of the most sensitive measuring range of the dosimeters (40 μR/Skt and 1.5 mR/Skt), the radiographic exposures were, in each case, repeated ten times within 5 minutes; the X-ray tube voltage was varied in steps between 77 and 125 kVp.

The dose measurements were repeated "in parallel" on a conventional X-ray unit under the identical geometrical radiographic conditions, using various film/screen combinations and the Alderson phantom. The results of these measurements are represented in Fig. 8.

Under standard conditions (125 kV), the following figures were obtained for the skin dose (on the surface of the phantom facing the radiation source) in the region of the abdomen:

Digital radiograph:
Size of field $512 \times 530\ mm^2$: $D = 3.0 \pm 0.2$ mR
Size of field $256 \times 270\ mm^2$: $D = 5.9 \pm 0.3$ mR

X-ray film ("plain view of the kidneys") standard film/screen combination, 125 kV, automatic exposure device:

Size of field $300 \times 400\ mm^2$: $D = 630 \pm 20$ mR.

1 Physikalisch-Technische Werkstätten Dr. Pychlau, Freiburg i. Br.

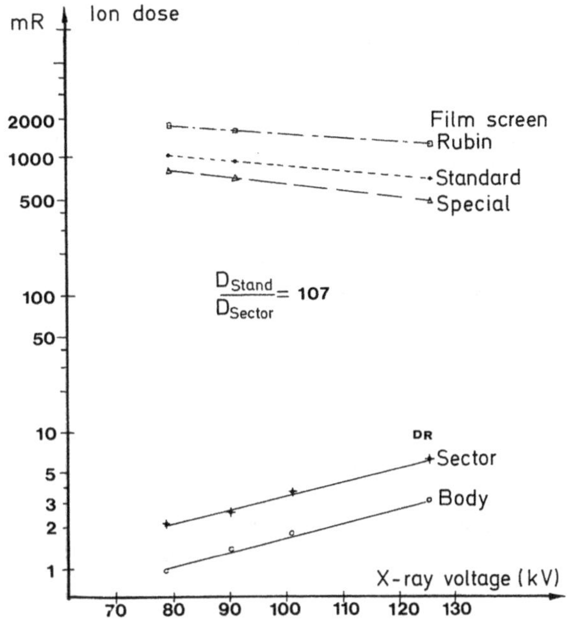

Fig. 8. Measurement of the ion dose in the Alderson phantom (abdomen) in the digital radiograph (*DR*) and in various film/screen combinations as a function of the X-ray tube voltage (kVp)

The contradictory relationship of the course of the dose with variation of the X-ray quantum energy in the digital radiograph and the film exposure, as revealed in Fig. 8, results from the constant, non-regulated emission of radiation in the digital radiograph, coupled with increased radiation absorption with reduction of the energy; in contrast, in the case of the conventional film radiograph, the automatic exposure device located on the side of the film compensates for the increased absorption of radiation of low quantum energy within the body by increasing the exposure, which leads to an increase in the skin dose.

The scattered radiation at the boundaries of the field show the course characteristic for the digital radiograph and occasioned by the strong collimation of the X-ray beam, with the – measured for the X-ray film image – very rapid drop-off in dose outside the exposure field.

These measurements show that, in the recording of digital radiographs that do not directly "involve" the gonads the *gonadal burden* is very small. It can be estimated that, at a distance of 50 mm between the gonads and the radiographic area in a man, a dose to the gonads of 100 μR (size of the field $256 \times 270\ mm^2$) or 40 μR ($512 \times 520\ mm^2$) results, the comparable figure for women being about 10 μR.

2.2 Spatial and Density Resolution

The spatial and density resolution of an imaging system characterize the quality and efficiency of such an apparatus. The objective of an image-transmission system must be to "handle" (process) and image a body on the object side as faithfully as possible. One criterion for the quality of the image transmission is the transformation of a *contrast* (*Stieve* 1966). In connection with imaging procedures, the term "contrast" may be understood to mean the difference between two or more object properties that represent objectifiable gradients – to be defined in detail – that can be assessed either by means of a measuring procedure or perceptually by an observer. Thus, for example, the eye can perceive steps of grey as a contrast between light and dark; in the case of the X-ray image, density contrasts can be converted to contrasts of blackening on a film, via a transfer function of an image-producing procedure.

The mathematical definition of contrast is not uniform. If there is a linear relationship between two "contrasting" parameters I_1 and I_2, the contrast K between them can be determined, for example, by the quotient:

$$K = \frac{I_1 - I_2}{I_1 + I_2}$$

All the definitions of contrast determined in this manner have in common that the maximum value of the contrast is given by $K = 1$, and the minimum value by $K = 0$ (when $I_1 = I_2$). This means that all contrasts can be described by a figure lying between 0 and 1 (0–100%).

The objective of an image-transmitting system should be to transmit a contrast within the object so as to produce this contrast as faithfully as possible in the image. Very frequently, the demonstration of a contrast between two magnitudes depends not merely on the contrast K between them within the object, but also upon the size of the object. A feature common to almost all image-producing procedures is that a small object with a marked contrast is more easily recognizable than an identical object with small contrast. Therefore, for the assessment of a transmission system, it is expediênt to vary the two parameters (size of the object and object contrast), in order, by recording a contrast-detail diagram, to investigate the efficiency of this procedure in comparison with other systems.

In order to carry out the necessary measurements, two separate setups are employed that permit:

1. The measurement of the spatial resolution under conditions of high contrast (determination of the smallest object size that can be visualized)
2. The measurement of the spatial resolution under conditions of low contrast (for the determination of the smallest visible contrast)

2.2.1 Spatial Resolution Under Conditions of High Contrast

In order to determine the smallest size of object that can be visualized by the digital radiographic technique, steel wires varying in diameter between 0.50 and 0.05 mm were affixed to a sheet. The contrast K vis-a-vis air, has the value of 1.

The evaluation of the radiography shows that with variation of the object direction and the size of the field, a resolution limit of $d = 0.15$ mm object diameter is achieved. The contrast recorded in the image, however, is considerably reduced, since the visualization of the thin object is effected in the 1×1.2-mm image "grid" of the radiograph, which is determined by the size of the detector and the X-ray pulse interval. As a result of the averaging of the 0.15-mm broad object, and the ambient air in the image-determining raster, a marked fictitious density enhancement of the object occurs in the image, resulting in a "partial-volume effect".

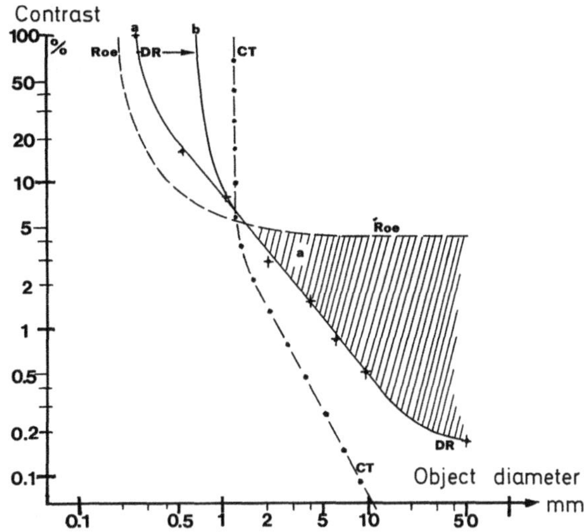

Fig. 9. Contrast-detail diagram for digital radiography (*DR*), standard X-ray film (*Roe*) and computerized tomography (*CT*). The curve *a* in *DR* marks the resolution of an individual object, and *b* the separability of small details. The hatched region *a* defines the region in which digital radiography proves superior to the conventional X-ray film

On account of the line and raster structure of the radiograph, the spatial separability of very small objects is reduced. If, for example, under a measuring magnifying glass, fine steel wires having a diameter of 0.50 mm are arranged and fixed in a row, with spacings varying between 0.20 and 1.0 mm, two of these high-contrast bodies can be separated in the image only when the spacing between them is at least 0.60 mm. With respect to the clinical evaluation of the digital radiograph, this limit of resolution is of greater significance than the minimum spatial resolution since, in a radiograph of a patient, details that need to be resolved are almost always contiguous (for example, the spongy structure in a bone).

2.2.2 Spatial Resolution Under Conditions of Low Contrast

In order to determine the spatial resolution under conditions of low contrast, a model comprising a Plexiglas body provided with a system of communicating channels, was developed. These connecting channels had a length of 60 mm and diameters varying between 1.0 and 6.0 mm; larger objects were investigated separately. In order to reproduce a situation comparable to that which is obtained when examining patients, the model was placed in a container filled to a depth of 200 mm with water, which represented the patient's body with its radiation scattering effect.

By filling the system of interconnecting channels with solutions of contrast material having different concentrations and known physical density [Urografin 76%, Urovison 58%, Rayvist 300 (Schering)], densities of between 1.418 and 1.000 g/cm^3 were produced, which represented density contrasts to polystyrene (ϱ= 1.180 g/cm^3), and water (ϱ= 1.000 g/cm^3 at 20 °C) of defined magnitude.

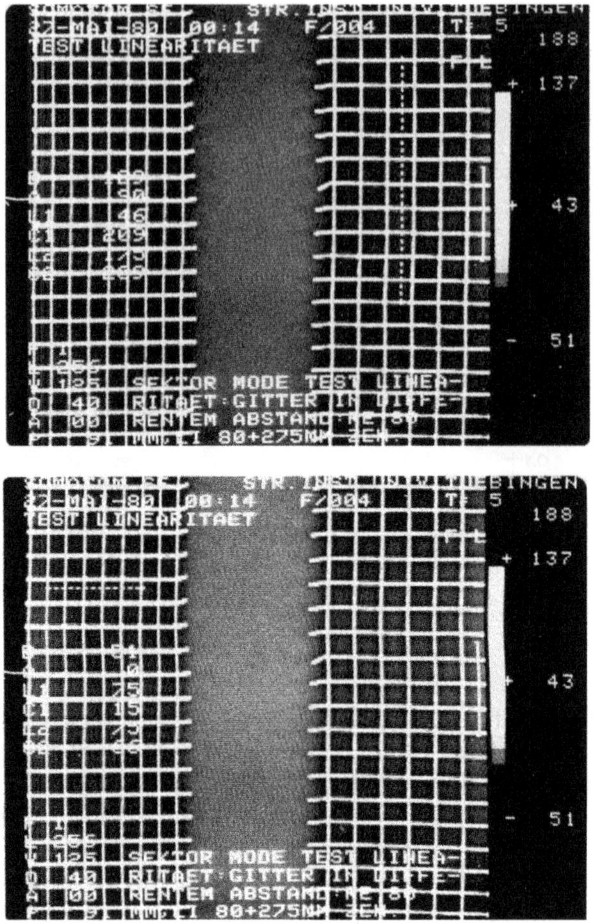

Fig. 10. Digital radiographs obtained of two identical measuring grids at different distances from the X-ray source

The production of digital radiographs of this model (phantom) while varying the parameters (size of the field, X-ray tube voltage, contrast material concentration and diameter of the object) permits the establishment of the contrast-detail diagram for the standard radiographic technique, as shown in Fig. 9. On the basis of model testing in the CT scanner and the X-ray film view, it is also possible to carry out comparative investigations. These can be obtained from the diagram.

It is shown (see Fig. 9) that in the case of small objects (up to about 1.5 mm in diameter) the conventional film radiograph is, with adequate contrast, clearly superior to both the digital radiograph and the computerized tomogram. For objects larger than about 2 mm in diameter, however, on account of the better density resolution (region a, Fig. 9), digital radiography is seen to be superior to the conventional film view. In the CT scan, an even greater density resolution can clearly be recognized. These advantages of the digital radiograph vis-a-vis the film radiograph are investigated in the clinical section.

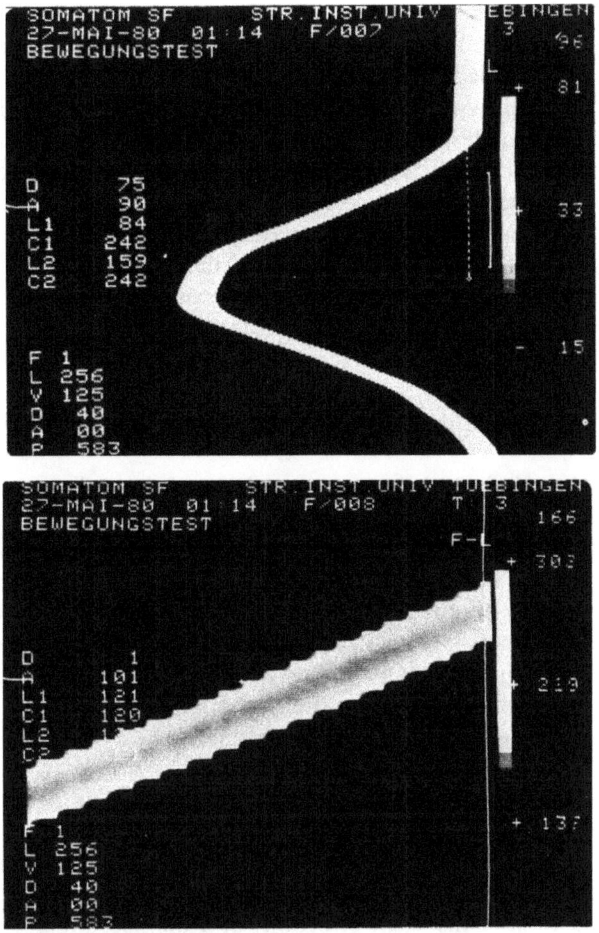

Fig. 11. Digital radiograph of the motion defined. The detail enlargement (*below*) shows the development of a stepped curve, as described in the text, which is brought about by the movement of the object and the pulsation of the X-ray beam

2.3 Linearity of the Image Transmission

In the case of digital radiography, the linearity of the image transmission is determined by the nature of the image production, which involves a different image build-up in the two coordinates of the radiograph. In the *transverse direction,* the data are "picked up" by the fan-shaped X-ray beam as in the case of the film radiography so that, in accordance with the "laws of radiation", objects are visualized on the detector plane in a computable geometrical projection that varies with the focal and film distance.

Along the longitudinal axis of the patient's body, thanks to the continuous movement of the patient, imaging is effected approximately in the central beam, so that, in the direction of the ordinate of the radiograph, no distortion of the projection occurs. This means, therefore, that in the direction of the abscissa an image of the object, linear in the direction of the ordinate, can be expected, in conformity with the "law of radiation".

In order to check this assumption, linear metal grids having a defined mesh size (0.5″) made of 1-mm thick wires were fixed at various distances, and radiographs made (Fig. 10). These images reveal the expected non-linearity in the direction of the abscissa, while along the oridinate a linearity of 2% resulted. For this reason, the measurement of distances and angles on the basis of the software is possible only when account is taken of the image transmission properties. Thus, in the transversal direction, the measurement of distances is valid only at an object distance of about 200 mm over the table top.

2.4 The Influence of Object Motion on Image Transmission

The relatively long exposure times of the radiograph (depending upon the radiographic format, 10 and 20 s), would suggest that movements of the object would lead to errors in the radiograph. At the beginning of this article, however, it was pointed out that, as a result of using pulsed X-radiation of 2 ms pulse duration, virtually no unsharpness due to physiological movements can arise. Maximal organ movements (velocity of the apex of the heart v (max) = 250 mm/s) give rise to an unsharpness of $\Delta s = v \times \Delta t = 250\ \mathrm{mm/s} \times 2\ \mathrm{ms} = 0.5\ \mathrm{mm}$.

This figure is below the threshold of detection in the contrast detail diagram in the presence of less than maximum contrast (Fig. 9).

If, during the exposure, the patient performs an active movement, a discontinuity of the image in the ordinate direction is to be expected. In order to test this assumption, movement of the object was simulated.

During the taking of the radiograph, a square-section ($30 \times 30\ \mathrm{mm}^2$) aluminium rail having a length L and fixed at one end was moved in the direction of the abscissa (transversal direction) at a defined angular velocity. From this combined translation-rotation movement, for each object point X (t) below the radiographic plane, the movement formula:

$$X(t) = v \cdot t \cdot \tan \omega t$$

resulted.

The digital radiograph of this object moved in the manner described shows the approximated tangential curve of each visualized object point (Fig. 11). At the same time, the development of steps in the moving object, caused by the pulsed X-ray emission become clear, although the object reveals no unsharpness. The step size (Fig. 11, detail enlargement) represents a measure for the velocity of the movement. At the interval period of 38 ms between two X-ray pulses (as delivered by the installation investigated here), the object had moved through 1 mm. This means that the object had a velocity of $v = \Delta s/\Delta t = 1\ \mathrm{mm}/38\ \mathrm{ms} = 26\ \mathrm{mm/s}$ in the lateral direction.

It can be shown that at a known distance of the object from the radiographic plane (detectors), for example, from the stepped curve of the heart contour, a kymographic motion analysis can become possible.

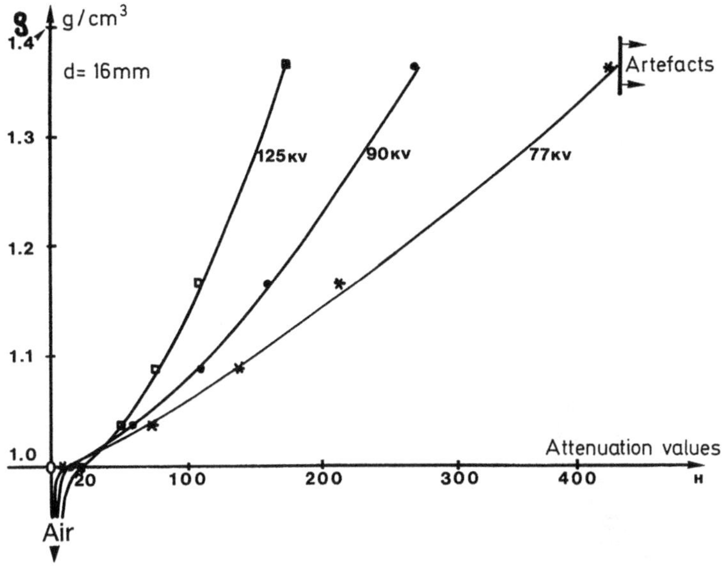

Fig. 12. Measurement of an identically sized object (attenuation value measurement) with variation of the object density, in the standard digital radiograph

2.5 Evaluation of Attenuation Measurements

The capability for carrying out attenuation measurements, as is made possible in the digital radiograph by the software taken over from CT, has only little practical value. Although in the measurement of absorption values employing the Hounsfield scale in test bodies of defined identical dimensions and varying density nonlinear correlations are found (Fig. 12), for the examination of patients these are of only little value. This is due on the one hand to the changes in measured values that occur during image reconstruction and which are not analysable, and, on the other, to the fact that in the superimposed images of the digital radiograph, only the product of the mass absorption coefficient μ, and the thickness of the object d, can be determined. In the absence of a knowledge of the thickness of the object, therefore, the product of these two parameters permits no conclusions to be drawn as to the integral attenuation of the body examined. At most, it permits a relative measurement in a comparison of the two sides, for symmetrical, transparent structures within the body (for example the lungs).

2.6 Errors and Artefacts

In the analysis of the most important artefacts and image errors that can occur in the digital radiograph, mention here shall be made only of those brought about by a too small number of quanta, and those that have their origin in the reconstruction algorithm. Imaging disturbances due to technical faults will not be discussed.

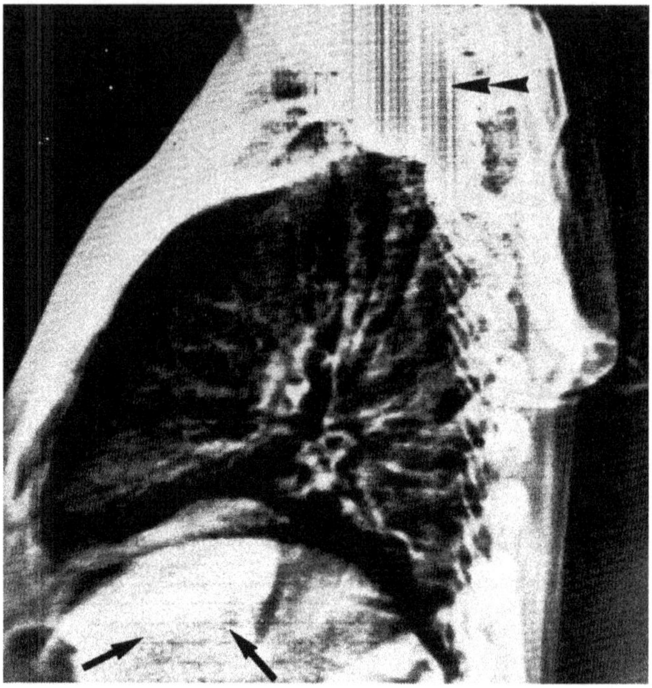

Fig. 13. Artefacts resulting from an inadequate signal-to-noise ratio: *arrow,* just measurable, but too small a signal (Moiré); *double arrow,* absent signal level

2.6.1 Artefacts Due to an Inadequate Number of Quanta

If the minimum number of quanta required in the detector for the production of an adequate signal-to-noise ratio is not achieved, imaging errors will occur within the radiograph that considerably impoverish the quality of the image or prevent the build-up of an image capable of interpretation. Since, in the equipment investigated, a relatively low number of quanta (and thus dose) are employed in the abdominal region or lateral views in the region of the shoulder girdle and pelvis in adipose patients, artefacts may occur due to an inadequate signal-to-noise ratio.

The gradation of the inadequate measured value level manifests in the radiograph in different ways:

1. A signal-to-noise ratio that is too low, but still measurable (Fig. 13): The useful signal is masked by the statistically scattered background quantum noise. The line structure on which measured signal components are superimposed is visualized as a moiré pattern.
2. No measurable signal-to-noise ratio: If the number of quanta "perceived" by the detector drops even further, an object-modulated useful signal is no longer picked up, and an image reconstruction is no longer possible. Merely statistically distributed photons are picked up ("perceived") and produce a picture, striped in the direction of the ordinate, which is due to the differing sensitivity of the detectors (artefacts induced by calibration).

3. Artefacts induced by calibration: As in the case of a too small, or absent, signal-to-noise ratio, artefacts can also occur when the measuring sensors have been inadequately calibrated. These then manifest slight variations in sensitivity which have to be compensated for by the series-connected amplifier. If this calibration is not carried out, the differences in sensitivity lead to differences in the identical measuring magnitude in the various detectors, and thus to the formation of detector-localized stripy artefacts in the direction of the longitudinal axis of the body (ordinate) (Fig. 13). The stripy artefact occurring in the image readily permits the determination of the faulty measuring sensor.

2.6.2 Artefacts Brought About by the Reconstruction Process

The reconstruction modality involving convolution of the measured value profile under standard conditions, with a low-pass function, leads to a marked edge-enhancement at the boundaries of an object having significantly different radiation absorption properties. If the attenuation differences are not too extreme, this mathematically differentiating edge enhancement gives rise to a visually "pleasant" emphasizing of the object boundary that is similar to the edge enhancement seen in xeroradiography. This marked edge enhancement, that comes about largely as a result of the "take-over" of the reconstruction algorithms from computerized tomographic convolution, can, however, lead to a marked degradation of the image impression, which can be compensated for only by adjusting the window setting, or by employing less strongly differentiating reconstruction functions. In the radiographs obtained under standard conditions, these edge effects, in particular the boundaries between heart and lungs, lungs and diaphragm, intestinal gas and gas-free abdomen, tissue and osteosynthetic material or chest wall and air, can give rise to such "empty zones" which, as also in attenuation measurements, lead to non-utilizable, "adulterated" values which have been induced since reconstruction.

Degradation of the image that can result from movements by the patient were mentioned in Sect. 2.4.

From the radiographic technique and the measured results obtained, the advantages and disadvantages of the new technology can be established, and these must be tested in clinical trials (*Foley* et al. 1979).

Advantages of digital radiography in comparison with conventional film radiography:

1. Very low exposure to the patient's body and the gonads to ionizing radiation
2. Extremely small scattered radiation component in the measured value recording (data acquisition)
3. High density and contrast resolving power
4. "Incorrect exposures" are not possible, provided there is an adequate number of photons
5. Simultaneous recording and reproduction of a large absorption value spectrum (that is, simultaneous hard and soft radiation radiography)
6. Rapid radiography of large areas of the body (for example, in polytraumatized patients)
7. Space-saving storage of the radiographs (electronic data carrier, no silver consumption)

8. Simple electronic manipulation of the image (for example, the production of subtraction radiographs, the measurement of attenuation values, distances, angles)
9. Distortion-free imaging in the longitudinal axis of the body
10. Additional apparatus-integrated examinations are also possible
11. Availability and transmission capability of the radiographs via cable or radio, to any site with data handling video devices
12. Further possibilities for the development of the system (improvement of spatial resolution, movement of the device instead of the patient, radiography with the patient standing)

At the present state of the technological art, the disadvantages of digital radiography vis-a-vis the conventional X-ray film radiographic technique may be summarized as follows:

1. Reduction of the spatial resolution of small objects having high contrast
2. In consequence of the relatively long exposure time for each radiograph, no dynamic (kinetic) studies are possible
3. The variability of the imaging format is restricted (this applies in particular to the imaging of small objects)
4. At present, radiographic capability is available only for recumbent patients, in the anteroposterior and lateral projections
5. All the technical possibilities can be fully utilized only at the evaluation equipment

3 Initial Clinical Experience with Digital Radiography

The assessment of a new diagnostic radiological procedure must be based on practical criteria. For this reason, more than 1500 radiographs were obtained and evaluated, all of which were "backed up" by conventional X-ray films, computerized tomographic scans and clinical information. The slow learning process in the handling of this innovative form of image representation and in the interpretation of the image, made it necessary that, initially, digital radiographs had to be obtained from already diagnosed pathological changes, so that a comparison and verification of the findings was possible. It was confirmed that, as a rule, the radiologist sees only that with which he is already familiar, and that for an assessment of an X-ray image "comparison" with the "memories" of images met with in the course of experience is often decisive.

The ability to make use of the advantages offered by this imaging procedure in the practical situation comes only with increasing experience, and as the examining physician learns to manipulate the grey-step control on the monitor and make full use of the electronic image manipulation capability.

Below, important normal findings and pathological states – usually in comparison with conventional film radiographs – are presented by way of example, to represent briefly the possibilities of the digital radiographic X-ray technique.

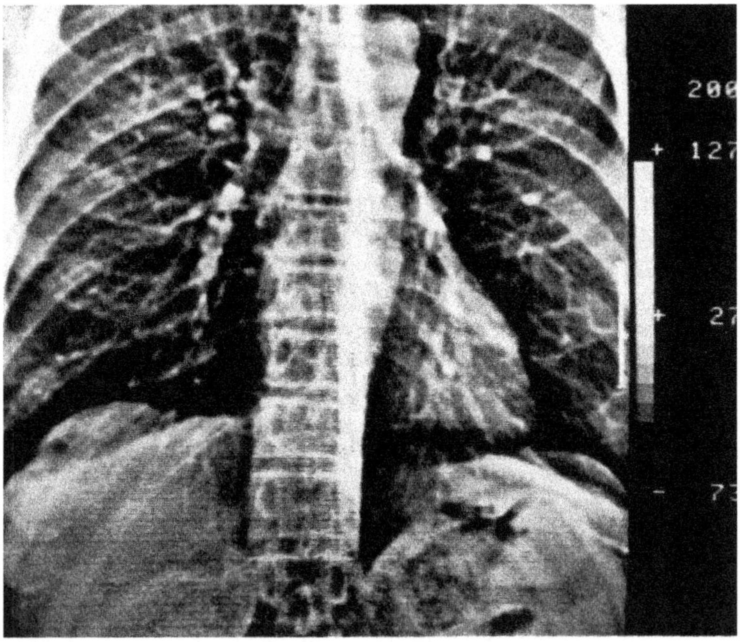

Fig. 14. Normal chest radiograph: the invariable format selection is a problem if the chest is too large. Equally good representation of the pulmonary structures, the structures of the heart, the vertebral column and the aorta, and also the pleural reflections

3.1 Digital Radiographic Diagnosis of the Chest

Usually, the radiograph of the chest has the format 256×270 mm^2, the entire trunk of large or adipose patients not always being completely imaged; the lack of a capability for a flexible modification of the radiographic format occasionally makes it necessary to obtain a second radiograph, the selection of a larger radiographic format usually not being recommended on account of the poorer spatial resolution. Conventionally, an anteroposterior view is obtained; the posteroanterior radiation beam can be employed in the present equipment only by repositioning the patient (in the prone position). Right and left lateral decubitus positions in conjunction with a lateral beam projection are just as easily obtainable as are side projections.

The heterogenous radiographic spectrum always permits the representation both of the skeletal structures, and of the soft parts; in the image examples shown, this variability cannot be demonstrated.

In the normal chest digital radiograph (Fig. 14) the mediastinal contours are simultaneously represented, including the trachea and main bronchi, the medial pleural reflections, the azygo-oesophageal line, the contour of the ascending and the descending aorta, and all parts of the heart.

The advantages of the superior contrast resolution can also be seen in the representation of the pulmonary structures in close proximity to the pleura; thus, the pulmonary blood vessels can be followed almost up to the lateral wall of the chest and also into the basal pulmonary recess behind the heart and liver.

The variability of the window setting means that various adjustments of the grey-step scale on the monitor are necessary, if the examining doctor wishes to make full use of the entire spectrum of diagnostic possibilities. This variable image representation requires considerable practice with respect to the establishment of the diagnosis, since the familiar reference and comparative structures representing important, sometimes, unconscious, criteria in the differential diagnosis of pathological changes in the conventional film radiograph (for example, the "hardness" of a circumscribed lesion: metastasis or tuberculoma) are lacking.

While, initially, prior to the evaluation of a digital radiograph, a conventional X-ray film view was needed to decide whether normal or pathological structures could be found in the digital radiograph, after some practice and the evaluation of about 400 digital chest radiographs, it became possible to establish a primary digital radiographic diagnosis and subsequently to compare it with the film view.

3.1.1 Diagnosis of the Lungs

The recognition of *circumscribed pulmonary lesions* in the conventional X-ray image depends upon their size, contrast and localization. Dense circumscribed lesions (tuberculomas) are not difficult to diagnose, while weakly contrasty lesions in close proximity to the pleura, and partially concealed by diaphragm or heart, can readily escape detection. In such cases, only the digital radiograph is capable of providing an improvement in the lesions "recognizability" (Figs. 15, 16). On account of the large differences in density between the circumscribed lesions and the pulmonary parenchyma, maximum contrast between the lesion and its surroundings is almost always present, so that, radiographically, a spatial resolution of 1–2 mm can be achieved; this means that the limiting diagnostic factor is not so much visualization of a detail, as, rather, the fact that recognition of an imaged detail is not unequivocal.

Intrapulmonary circumscribed lesions permit limited differential diagnostic evaluation with respect to the substrate of the lesion, on the basis of attenuation measurements, provided that, in comparison with the surrounding tissue, characteristic deviations from the normal attenuation ranges occur (for example, bronchiectasis and cysts, or calcified circumscribed lesions).

Pulmonary vessels can – sometimes in contrast to the film view – be followed right up into the periphery, and thus, in the digital radiograph, provide a basis for suspecting pulmonary congestion when the clinical picture does not exclude such a possibility. Dilated peripheral and central blood vessels, for example, in the case of a mitral stenosis, can, accordingly, just as readily be detected. Moreover, the thickened peripheral alveolar septa (Kerly lines) can also be detected radiographically in chronic pulmonary congestion.

Diffuse pulmonary diseases can be visualized on the basis of the increase in density that characterize them (Fig. 17). It may be expected that both interstitial and also alveolar exudation (for example in the case of pulmonary oedema) will also be diagnosable in the digital radiograph.

3.1.2 Pleural Changes

On account of the recognizability of the medial and basal pleural reflections in the digital radiograph, displacements of these structures are usually easier to interpret in the digital than in the conventional film radiograph.

Both medial and lateral extending and encapsulated *pleural effusions* can, radiographically, just as readily be detected and differentiated from a pneumothorax (Fig. 18). In contrast, in the recumbent radiographic position, small infrapulmonary effusions may present merely as a minimal density elevation, and thus require a second exposure with the patient in a lateral position. In consequence of the edge-enhancing effect in the digital radiograph, which is prevalent in the "transitional region" diaphragm/lungs, small reductions in transparency can, however, easily be overlooked.

3.1.3 Mediastinum

The digital radiograph of the chest routinely covers important mediastinal structures and contours:

1. The ascending and descending aorta
2. The left medial pleural reflection
3. The azygo-oesophageal line and the azygos vein
4. The trachea, together with the two main bronchi, occasionally also central sections of the lobular bronchi
5. The contour of the heart with kymographic marginal step formation.
6. The oesophageal lumen following Gastrografin or barium sulphate swallowing
7. Not regularly: the anterior mediastinal reflection, together with the pulmonary ligament of the superior pleuro-oesophageal recess
8. Superpositioning by the supraspinal ligament connecting the spinous processes of the thoracic vertebral bodies.

In these structures the characteristic pathologic changes can be detected, for example, a broadening of the upper part of the mediastinum due to an *aortic aneurysm* (Fig. 19) with elimination or displacement of the aortic contour, through a *lymphoma* or a retrosternal *struma* that brings about a constriction and a displacement of the trachea.

Impressions of the trachea or the parts of the bronchus proximal to the carina, due to the presence of a tumour, can often be just as reliably detected radiographically, as with blurring tomography (Fig. 20).

Displacements of the pleurae, as can, for example, occur in *mediastinal prolapse* (Fig. 21) or in *infradiaphragmatic mediastinal lymphoma,* can usually be just as reliably detected by means of digital radiography, as with conventional radiography of the vertebral column.

An adequate digital radiographic representation of the *oesophagus* is not possible, on account of the fact that the spatial resolution is not adequate for a detailed assessment of the mucous membrane. Only larger lesions, tumours, fistulae and diverticula can be demonstrated, with the aid of swallowing of undiluted Gastrografin.

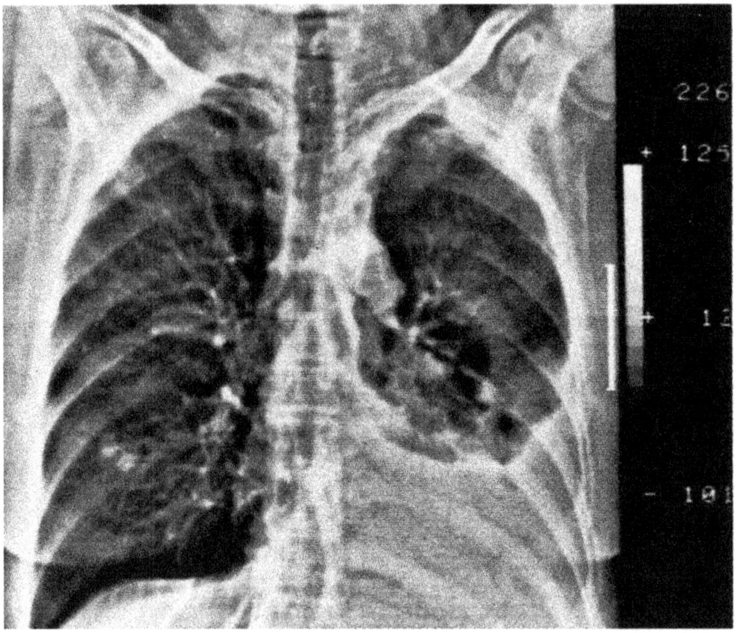

Fig. 15. Extending pleural effusion on the *left,* two pulmonary metastases in the right lower field and a further metastasis in the left middle field

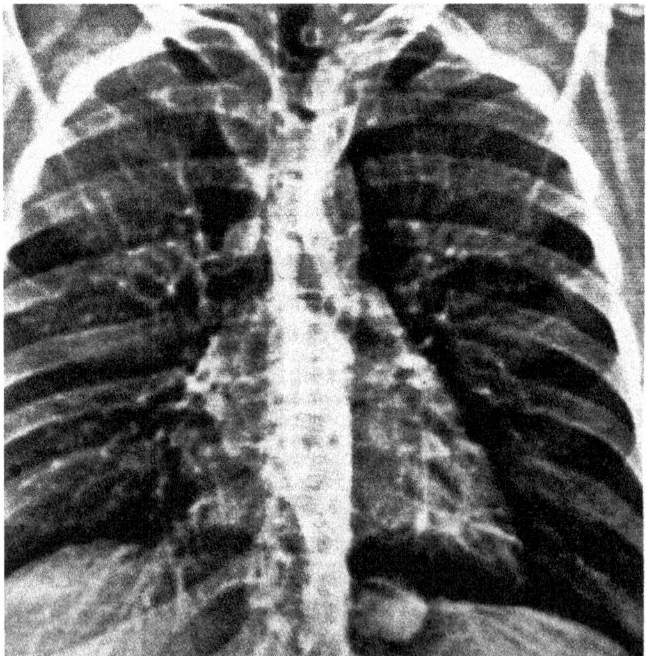

Fig. 16. Retrocardial metastasis from a seminoma in the posterior diaphragmatic recess

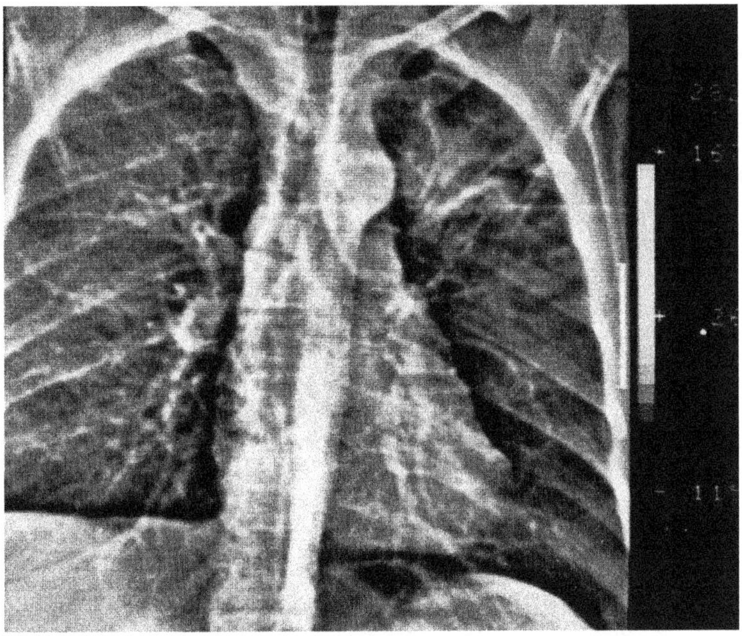

Fig. 17. Pneumonia in the upper field of the left lung

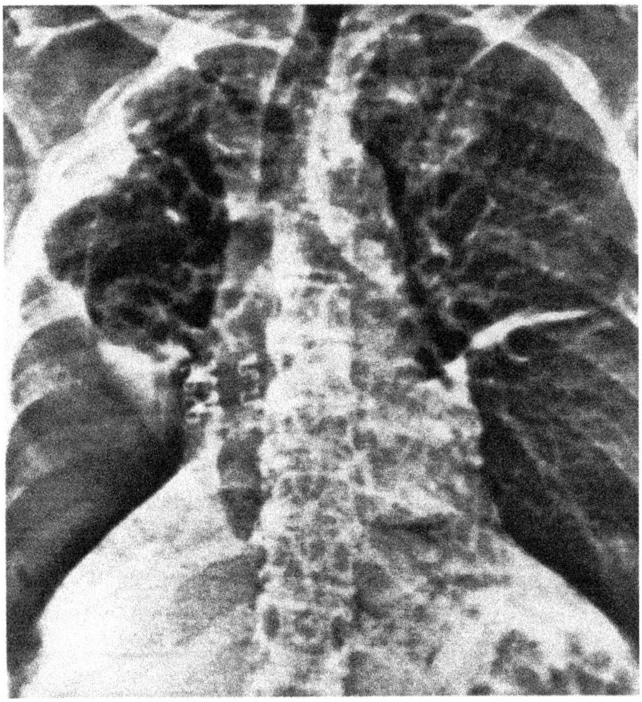

Fig. 18. Encapsulated seropneumothorax of the lower lobe of the right lung subsequent to recurrent pleural punctures

a 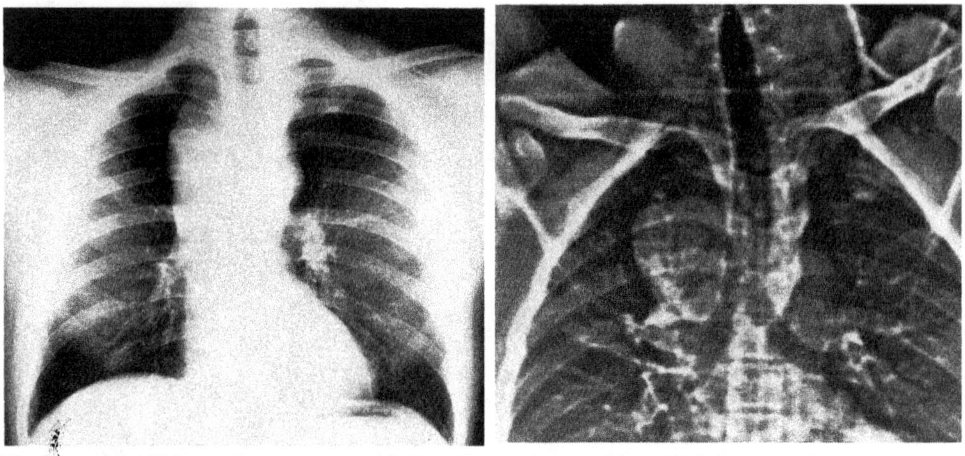 b

Fig. 19. **a** Syphilitic aortic aneurysm with invasion of the brachiocephalic trunk. Chest view in the erect patient. **b** Digital radiograph of the same patient. The absence of any narrowing of the trachea is well documented. With the modified window setting, the invasion of the brachiocephalic trunk is also clearly represented

a 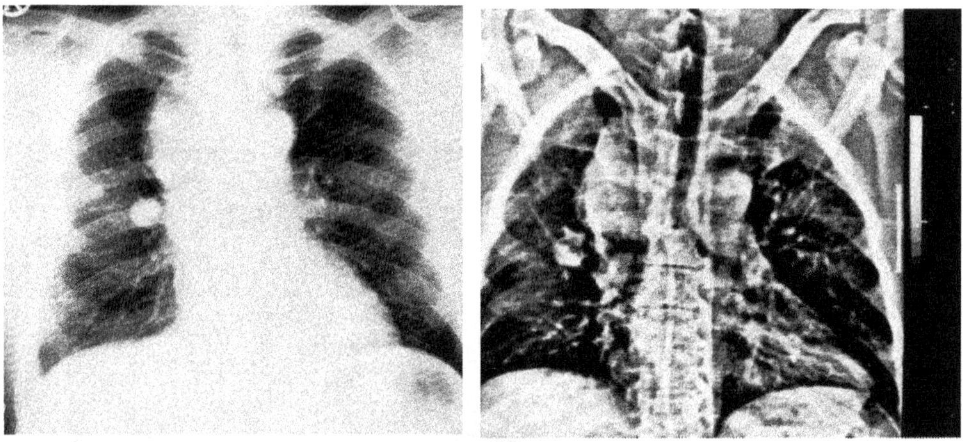 b

Fig. 20 a, b

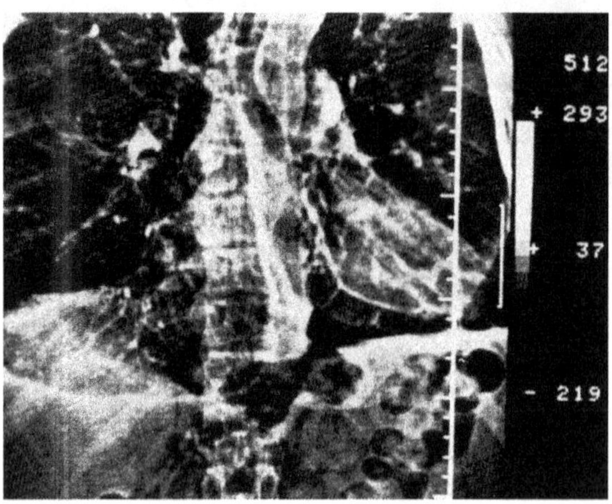

Fig. 21

3.1.4 Non-Contrast Examination of the Heart

Both the *heart* and the great blood vessels can be visualized by means of digital radiography just as readily as with conventional film radiography. There are, however, two important differences:

1. In view of the fact that the digital radiograph is obtained with the patient recumbent, the silhouette of the heart cannot be compared with that seen in the standard conventional film obtained with the patient standing
2. Owing to the long exposure time of 10 s, the cardiac contour is represented kymographically (see Sect. 2.4)

As a result of the movement of the patient's body – which, in the case of the equipment investigated here, was a constant 25 mm/s – this kymographic analysis, however, permits the study of only a few heart beats (four to six) so that, as a result, useful information about the motility of the myocardium is usually not possible. Here, the high-frequency "chronogram", the principle of which is described in Sect. 3.4, might possibly provide new details.

In the digital radiograph, almost always the entire silhouette of the heart, including the parts of the organ on which the diaphragm and vertebral column shadows are superimposed, is represented. This means that a complete assessment of the cardiac configuration is possible; in presenting cardiac pathology, for example, a ventricular enlargement or an enlarged atrial "core" shadow, the diagnosis can be easier than in the conventional film radiograph (Fig. 22).

3.2 Digital Radiographic Assessment of the Abdomen and Pelvis

The plain abdominal view obtained with the patient in the supine position serves to assess the soft tissue shadows of the parenchymatous organs, and also the skeletal structures. Using digital radiography, it is almost always possible to identify the liver, spleen, psoas muscles and the urinary bladder, together with the skeleton and the muscular abdominal wall, while the delimitation of the kidney contour is, owing to the superimposition of the gas-filled colon, in many cases, difficult (*Katragadda* et al. 1979). With the aid of the edge-enhanced, in part exaggerated, image reconstruction of the "transition" colonic wall-abdomen, for the identification of the kidneys, the attempt should always be made, by adjusting the window setting, to visualize all sections of the organ; to manage this with any degree of

Fig. 20. a A view of the thorax in the erect patient, showing a central bronchial carcinoma on the *right,* located at the origin of the upper-lobe bronchus, and atalectasis. A hilar metastasis can be seen on the right. **b** The same patient as in Fig. 20 a; now, both the narrowing of the distal part of the trachea caused by the tumour and also the impression effect on the left main bronchus caused by the carina lymph node can be recognized. The right bronchial trunk, which is almost completely enclosed by the tumourous growth, can no longer be seen; in contrast, the right pleural reflection and the contour of the vena cava can still be delimited

Fig. 21. Mediastinal prolapse, on the *right,* clearly recognizable despite the superimposed diaphragm and cardiac shadows. In addition, bronchiectasis, located retrocardially on the *left*

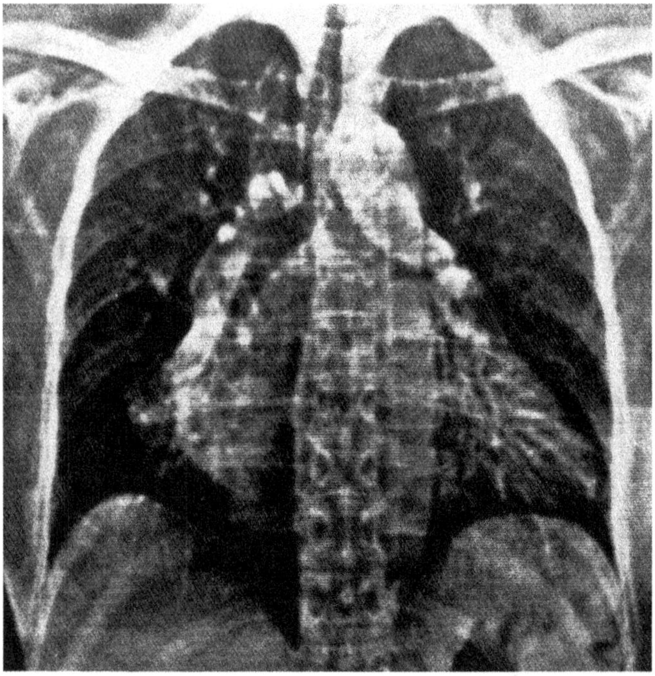

Fig. 22. Combined mitral pathology, predominantly mitral stenosis with considerable broadening of the carina, representing manifestations of dilation of the left atrium. With adjustment of the window setting the lung structure can be assessed

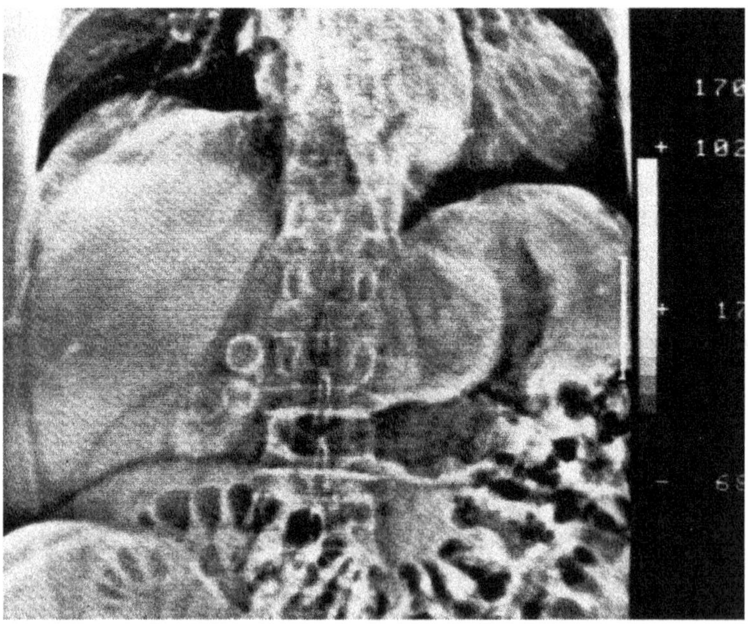

Fig. 23. Multiple gallbladder concrements showing circular calcification. The liver, the right kidney and the fundus and antrum of the stomach are all well delimited

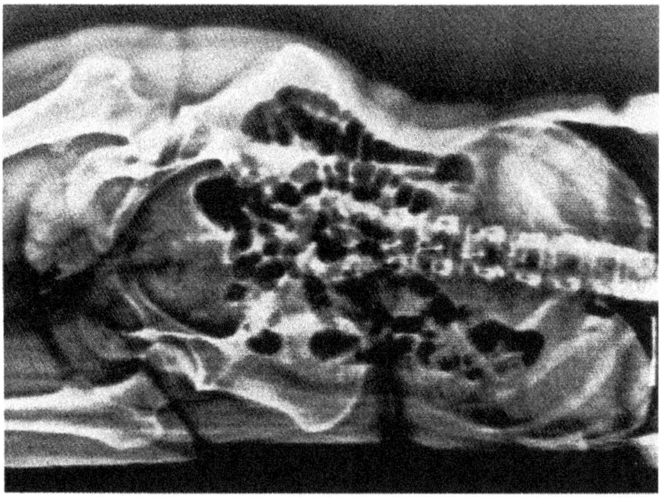

Fig. 24. Abdominal view with the patient in the left-lateral position (body mode): the normal, air-containing intestinal structures are readily distinguishable from the muscular abdominal wall and the diaphragm

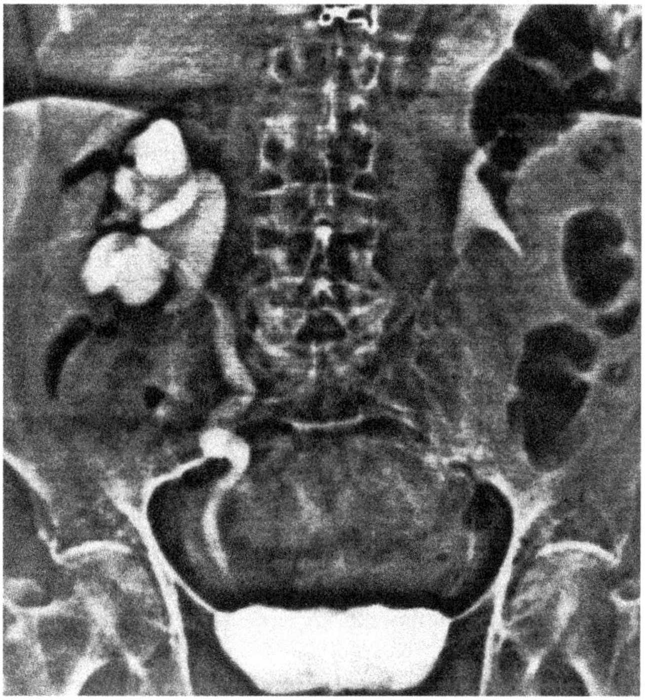

Fig. 25. Hydronephrosis on the *right*, with dilatation of the right ureter, showing perivesical scar formation after the surgical removal of a carcinoma of the body of the uterus

reliability, however, is not always possible. Dual energy subtraction radiography perhaps may solve this problem in the future.

Pathological non-contrast shadows such as those due to concrements (Fig. 23) and calcifications, as also tumour shadows, can readily be represented, in the same way as in the conventional non-contrast kidney film, since, in consequence to high density resolution, even small calcified biliary or renal concrements can be detected (*Lawson* et al. 1980). A particular advantage of the digital radiographic abdominal examination is that faulty exposures – which in conventional film radiography are something of a problem in this region on account of the high gonadal burden – are not possible.

The non-contrast digital radiograph of the abdomen in the left-lateral decubitus position, as is frequently required, for example, in patients with acute abdomen, would appear particularly favourable. "Free" air, or localized levels in the small or small intestine in patients with mechanical occlusion or local or general bowel atonia, is, on account of the high-contrast representation (Fig. 24) easier to diagnose in the digital radiograph than in the corresponding conventional radiograph. Here, too, the spatial resolution suffices to make it possible to detect fine "crescents" of air at the abdominal wall, which, particularly in the case of adipose patients, owing to the extremely high scattered radiation component and the resulting reduction in contrast, can readily escape detection in a conventional film.

3.2.1 The Use of Contrast Materials

As already mentioned in the case of the oesophagus, the use of contrast materials to opacify the gastrointestinal tract has only little significance for digital radiography, since the spatial resolution is not adequate to permit the visualization of mucosal relief and very small lesions. Equally disadvantageous is the fact that, owing to the long exposure times, it is not possible to produce fluoroscopic "spotfilms", so that the usefulness of contrast media in the bowel remains restricted. Although larger space-consuming processes such as diverticula can also be detected in the digital radiograph, the reliability and completeness of such an examination can, at best, be applied to patients with large lesions such as a tumour-induced stenosis; it appears reasonable for example only for the localization for radiotherapeutic purposes.

At present, the use of angiographic and cholegraphic contrast materials in digital radiography also has little value, since a fine interpretation of very small details such as, for example, the calyceal system in the kidneys, or the extrahepatic bile ducts, cannot be performed with adequate resolution, and unclear findings caused by overlapping phenomena cannot be further clarified by using blurring tomographic techniques.

Larger changes in the kidneys, ureters and urinary bladder, in contrast, can also be detected in the digital radiograph, so that this technique might be employed, for example, for the follow-up of a backup of urine, with the aim of reducing the radiation exposure, in a child, or during a pregnancy. Thus, a dilatation of the pelvicalyceal system of the kidney due to backup of urine, or inflammatory processes (Fig. 25), can readily by demonstrated; hereby, the contrast medium requirement is, thanks to the high density resolution, lower than in the case of conventional film radiography.

Thus, for example, for a representation of the kidneys, about 100 ml of a 30% nephrographic medium are usually sufficient.

Summarizing, therefore, primary diagnostic examinations of the kidneys and the efferent urinary tract, or of the efferent biliary ducts, cannot be considered tasks for digital radiography.

For the digital radiographic *representation of blood vessels* employing "angiographic" contrast materials, the following points may be made:

1. On account of the high density resolution, smaller quantities and lower concentrations of the contrast medium than those required by conventional radiographic examinations usually suffice (*Brody* et al. 1980).
2. On account of the long exposure times, a high concentration of contrast medium must be maintained within the blood vessels for a relatively long period (use of isoosmolar substances).
3. The integrated software readily permits the production of subtraction views after radiography; the long exposure times, however, rarely permit the production of identical radiographs prior to and following the administration of contrast medium.
4. On account of the reduced spatial resolution, minute vascular changes (as seen in, for example, Raynaud's disease) cannot be reliably detected in the digital radiograph.

By way of example, a number of possibilities may be mentioned:

Phlebographic examinations of the lower or upper extremities (Fig. 26) are, provided that adequate fixation is observed, possible, with adequate resolution, for subtraction techniques, so that the diagnosis of a thrombosis of the greater veins can be established with a relatively small amount of contrast medium (for example, 20 ml of a 30% angiographic contrast medium).

Transvenous angiography, as propagated by *Stenberg* et al. (1959), in conventional radiography, and by *Kramann* (1978) for xeroradiography of the extremities, would also appear, in the light of our own experience, a suitable technique for digital radiography, where it might be used as survey arteriography. Here, again, however, a particular disadvantage is the long exposure time needed to obtain a digital radiograph, that, in turn, requires a lengthy vascular opacification and, in addition, in consequence of the varying circulatory times of the blood, an individual "tailoring" of the moment of exposure (*Hübener* and *Klott* 1980). The production of subtraction views also remains a particular problem since, as a rule, it cannot be expected that the patient will remain immobile for two examinations. The subtraction view is, however, very desirable for keeping down the amount of intra-arterial contrast material required. The computer-controlled fluoroscopic units, based on rapid subtraction, which permit transvenous arteriography as digital fluoroscopy imaging or digital vascular imaging, have a "seconds rhythm", and can thus much more readily image the phase of arterial contrast material inflow after intravenous administration, and also better eliminate small movements of the patient, which would appear possible at the present time with digital radiography. On the other hand, the considerably superior contrast resolution of the digital

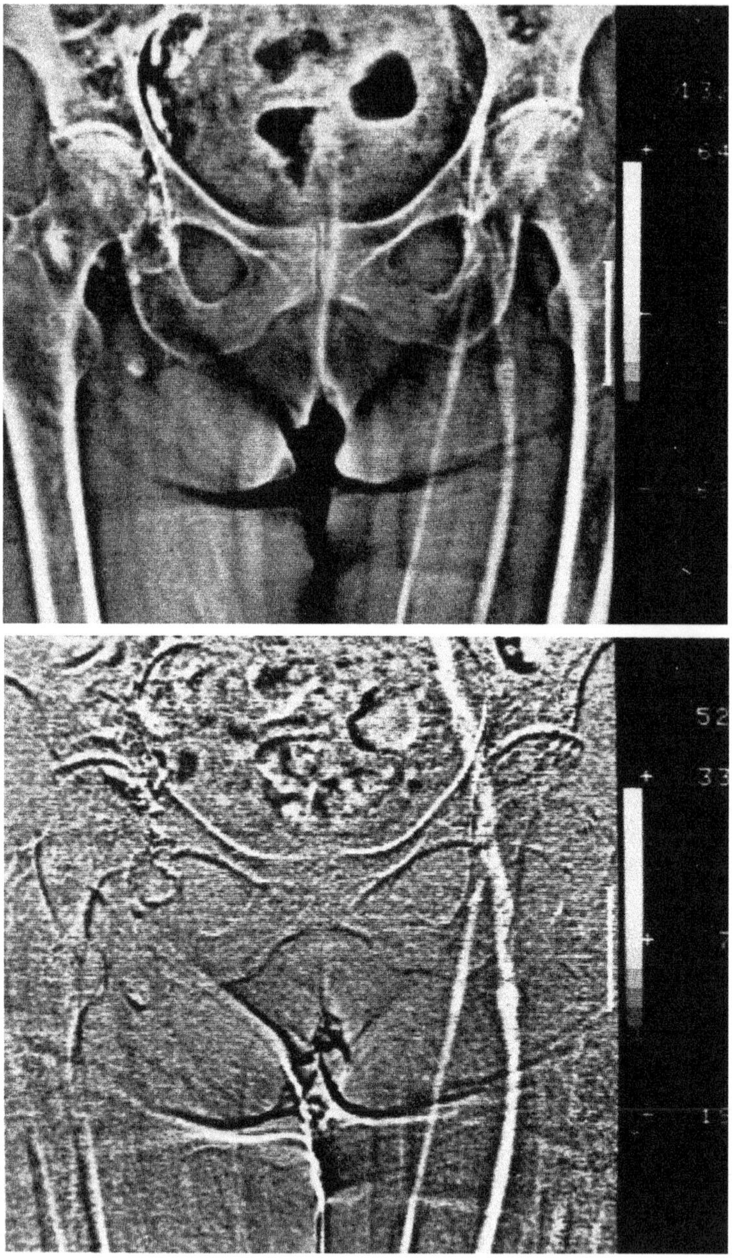

a

b

Fig. 26. a Phlebography of the left leg following the injection of 20 ml Rayvist 235. The iliac vein is hardly discernible. **b** Subtraction view obtained after subtracting a non-contrast view obtained prior to the administration of contrast material to give the view shown in Fig. 26 a. The iliac vein is now better recognized; a valve can be seen in the femoral vein radiograph vis-a-vis the digital fluoroscopy procedure must be considered a major advantage. A feature common to both procedures is the low radiation burden for the patient.

As our own initial experiments have shown, pulsations in the vicinity of the larger arteries, displacements of air-containing structures overlapping the blood vessels and the edge-enhanced radiograph reconstruction, represent further major disturbing factors for vascular imaging. Further detailed investigations, that also include the use of non-ionic contrast materials – which, on account of the fact that they remain within the vessels for longer periods, make them appear particularly suitable for this type of blood vessel representation – should soon permit an answer to the question as to whether, with this type of image representation, it will be possible to carry out an adequate transvenous arteriography of the great vessels. The dual energy subtraction radiography seems to become the other way to solve this problem.

3.3 Skeletal Examinations

The reduction of spatial resolution of digital radiography, in particular with high-definition (fast) film/screen combinations, lowers the value of this imaging procedure in the diagnostic examination of lesions affecting the bones. Particularly, very fine changes in the structure of the spongy bone, fractures without any displacement of the fragments, or fissures, are – in analogy to the results of the contrast detail diagram – not visualized in the radiograph with any degree of reliability.

Major bony changes, for example, fractures that require urgent treatment, can, however, readily be detected with digital radiography. In particular the rapid visualization of large areas of the body in polytraumatized patients, thus makes it possible to decide whether a primary surgical or a conservative intervention is required, within only a few minutes (with a radiographic time for the entire body of about 1 min). In a detailed investigation, *Ayella* (1978) pointed out that, in polytraumatized patients, the usually time-consuming X-ray examinations not infrequently led to serious delays in the primary care given to these patients; at that time, indeed, this study stimulated efforts to develop faster X-ray diagnostic procedures, which, in turn led to the digital radiographic imaging device developed by *Stein* (1975). In a study involving the examination of 18 massively traumatized patients using a digital radiological system, *Curtis* (1979) was able to show that all the major abnormalities in need of emergency treatment were recognized. He drew particular attention to the short exposure time (microdose), the large field of examination, the consistency of the exposure (no repeat examinations were necessary), the capability for simultaneous viewing of the image at various sites, the fact that image motion does not destroy the useful quality of the image, and the fact that low radiation scatter permits the attending personnel to be present during the examination (for example, for ventilation of the patient).

3.3.1 Diagnostic Examination of the Head

The radiographic diagnostic examination of the head (*Baker* 1981) is restricted to bony defects and fractures that need to have a minimum size of about 5 mm in

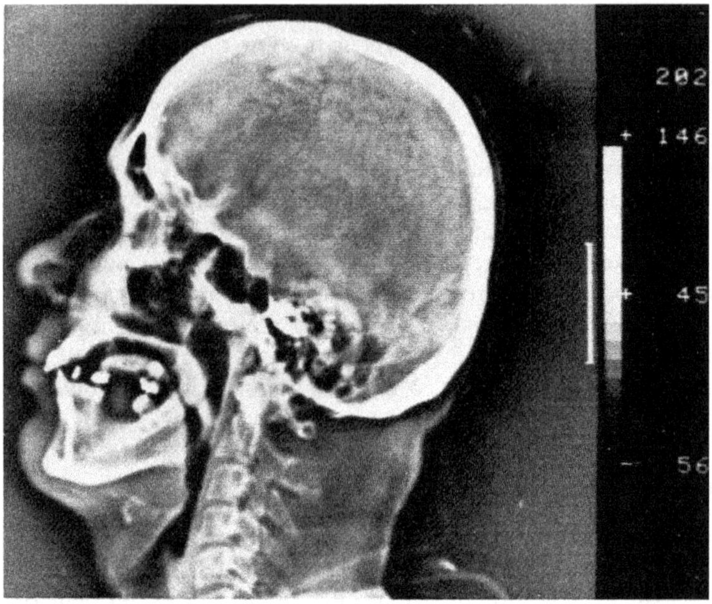

Fig. 27. A radiograph showing a lateral view of the head. In addition to the bony structure, the peripheral soft tissues and also the pharynx are particularly well represented

diameter or – in the case of fractures – the presence of a "step" of 2–3 mm, in order to be reliably detected. A considerable advantage in this respect is the simultaneous visualization of soft tissue abnormalities, which in the conventional film radiograph can be reproduced only with a strongly collimated image format capable of reducing the scattered radiation, but at the same time reducing the energy of the radiation beam. The normal soft part silhouette can also readily be imaged (Fig. 27), an advantage which, for example, can be of considerable relevance for the radiotherapeutic treatment planning in the case of tumours of the facial skeleton.

The skull can be visualized with a variety of projections by repositioning the head of the patient, even with the setting of the radiographic device in only two planes.

As in the case of the conventional X-ray film, in addition to the soft parts, the structures of the facial skeleton and the cranium can also be represented with good resolution. In consequence of the high contrast, the cranium appears radiographically more transparent and, in the marginal structures, not subjected to excessive radiation. The high level of density discrimination of the radiograph permits a better differentiation of cranium attenuation brought about by vascular changes than is possible in the conventional film radiograph. Even with considerable overlapping of soft tissues, bony defects (Fig. 28) can be represented, while fissures in the base of the skull will probably escape radiographic detection.

3.3.2 Examination of the Vertebral Column

The most important application at present of digital radiography in conjunction with the computerized tomography scanner is considered to be the possibility of

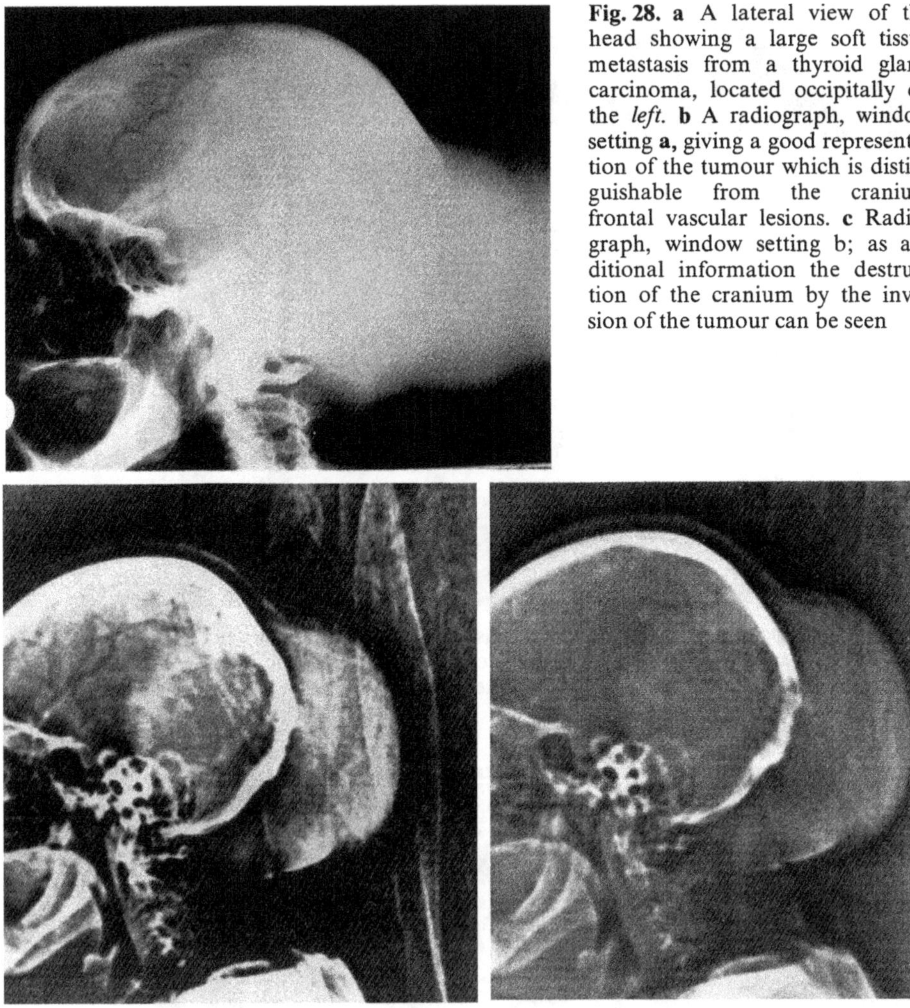

Fig. 28. a A lateral view of the head showing a large soft tissue metastasis from a thyroid gland carcinoma, located occipitally on the *left*. **b** A radiograph, window setting **a,** giving a good representation of the tumour which is distinguishable from the cranium frontal vascular lesions. **c** Radiograph, window setting b; as additional information the destruction of the cranium by the invasion of the tumour can be seen

a b c

being able to locate accurately the CT transversal layers parallel to the vertebral bodies, or to the intervertebral discs, a possibility that is indispensable for an adequate investigation of the vertebral canal (Fig. 29). Here, the angular measurement in the radiography offers ideal preconditions for the correct positioning of the gantry of the computerized tomographic scanner. In the anteroposterior beam projection, scoliotic vertebral column changes, as well as degenerative structural changes, can be diagnosed and, wherever necessary, taken into account for the setting of the transversal slice. A number of investigations dealing with the possibilities of computerized tomographic diagnostic examination of the vertebral column indicate that computerized tomography, in conjunction with the digital radiograph, will, in the future, make most myelographic examinations superfluous.

While, for the assessment of the vertebral canal, the CT scan is indispensable, digital radiography *alone* is able to visualize a number of conditions affecting the

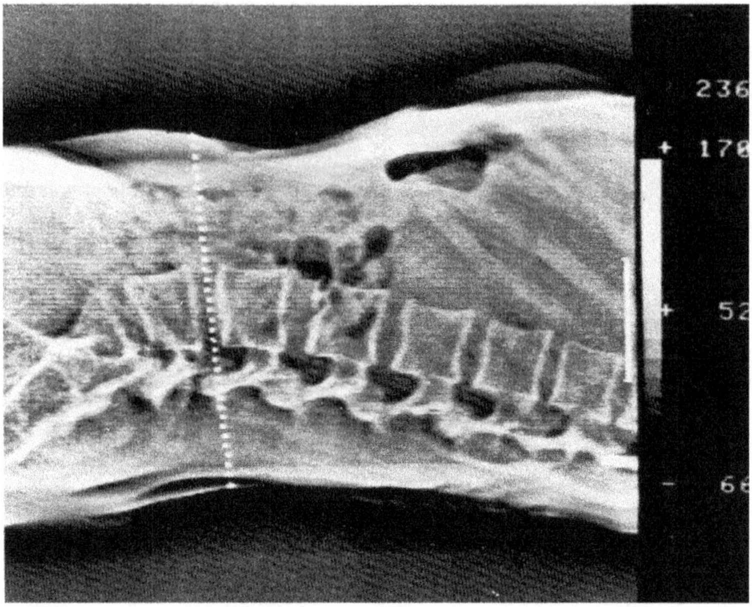

Fig. 29. Lateral view of the abdomen to visualize the lumbar vertebral column in a CT examination of the vertebral canal (prolapse of the intervertebral disc). Measurement of the tilt of the intervertebral space to establish the setting of the CT slice (*dotted line*)

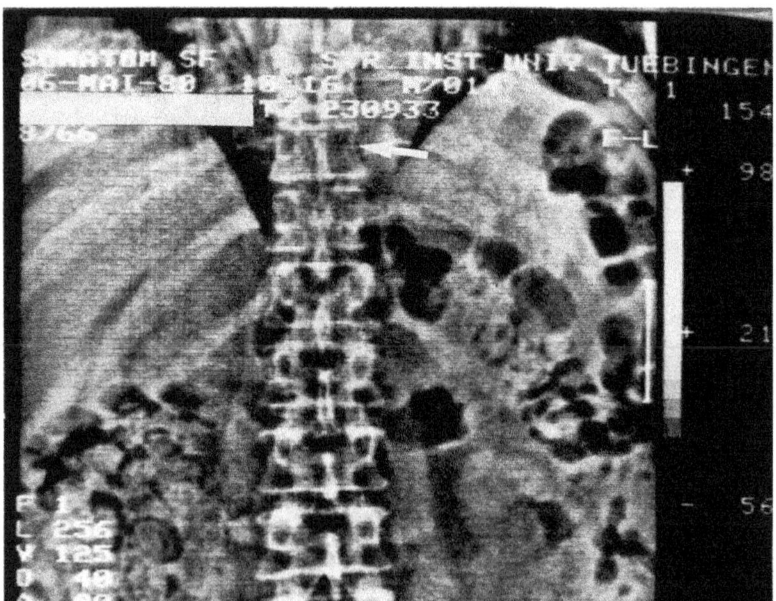

Fig. 30. Elimination of the "root" of the left vertebral arch, of the X thoracic vertebra (*arrow*), by an osteolytic metastasis of a hypernephroid carcinoma

vertebral column; as already mentioned, also in the case of digital radiographs of the chest or abdomen the vertebral column can also be visualized with appropriate modification of the window settings on the monitor. The "fixed" dose output of the X-ray tube in the equipment available at present, however, at too small a number of quanta, and too small a signal-to-noise ratio, does not always permit artefact-free and satisfactory image quality.

Radiographically detectable are degenerative changes, such as spondylosis, a reduction in the "height" of the vertebral body, for example, in cases of superior vertebral plate rupture, and also metastatic defects (for example, osteolytic destruction of a "root" of a vertebral arch, Fig. 30). Postoperative bone defects, such as window lesions, can be recognized without any difficulty, while discrete changes, which can usually be clarified only with the aid of conventional "blurring tomography", will probably escape reliable and consistent detection in the digital radiograph.

An assessment of the calcium salt content on the basis of the subjective picture "impression" is something of a problem, since the window setting of the video monitor makes it very difficult to quantify the density. From basic principles, however, on account of the high density discrimination, it may be expected that, with standardized radiographic procedures *and* a defined grey-step setting, it should become possible to assess the integral calcium salt content of the body to the same degree as is possible in the conventional film radiograph.

3.3.3 Diagnostic Examination of the Soft Tissues

Owing to the high-contrast radiographic technique, the soft part "covering" of the body head and extremities of the patient can be imaged better with digital radiography than with conventional radiography. In addition to the contours of the body – owing, in particular, to the edge-enhanced image reconstruction – the skin, subcutaneous fat and musculature in the "marginal" parts of the body are represented. In the presence of an adequate fat content, bundles of muscles can also be demarcated one from the other.

The usefulness of the digital radiograph in the diagnostic examination of the soft parts – which has to be individually "set-up" for each exposure – is probably to be seen in the improved detectability of pathological substances (calcifications, non-metallic foreign bodies).

In addition, such soft tissue changes as, for example, tumourous infiltration (Fig. 31) can be readily assessed in their localization and extent, and correctly assigned to the skeletal section.

3.4 High-frequency Transmission Radiography of a Narrow Transversal Slice Through the Body ("Chronogram")

The usual radiographic modality of the digital radiograph involves the movement of the patient beneath the imaging unit at a defined, constant speed, while the X-ray tube emits X-ray pulses at regular (equal) intervals. If, however, the patient is *not moved,* a rapid sequence of X-ray pulses leads to the transmission of a single

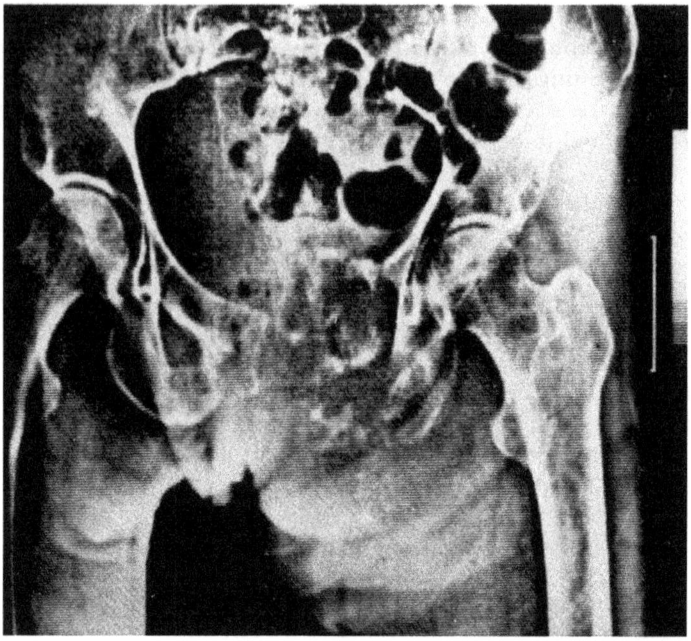

Fig. 31. Massive destruction of the left pubic and ischium bones with a large soft tissue tumour

slice through the patient's body. If, in this slice, which, in the case of the equipment investigated here is 8 mm in width, temporal changes in the attenuation values occur, these changes can be detected with the radiographic arrangement described. Such time-variable changes might, for example be:

1. Pulsation of the heart and blood vessels
2. Respiratory movements
3. Movements of the body
4. Contrast material flow

These parameters can modulate the transmission signal if this signal is repeated at a frequency that permits the detection of the changes in the velocity of the object under study.

In consequence of the high pulse repetition rate (pulsation sequence) of the X-ray generator of up to 50 impulses per second, correspondingly numerous transmission profiles can be recorded per unit of time. For the representation of these data, it has proved expedient to "line up" the sequentially recorded profiles in the ordinate direction on the television monitor screen, so that, here, the ordinate of the television image is allocated to the time axis, while, in the digital radiograph, it is "responsible" for representing the longitudinal axis of the body.

Since, in the case of the monitor employed as standard equipment, a television image is made up of 256 lines, an identical number of transmission profiles can be visualized. At an X-ray pulse repetition rate of, for example, 50 per second, this

a
b
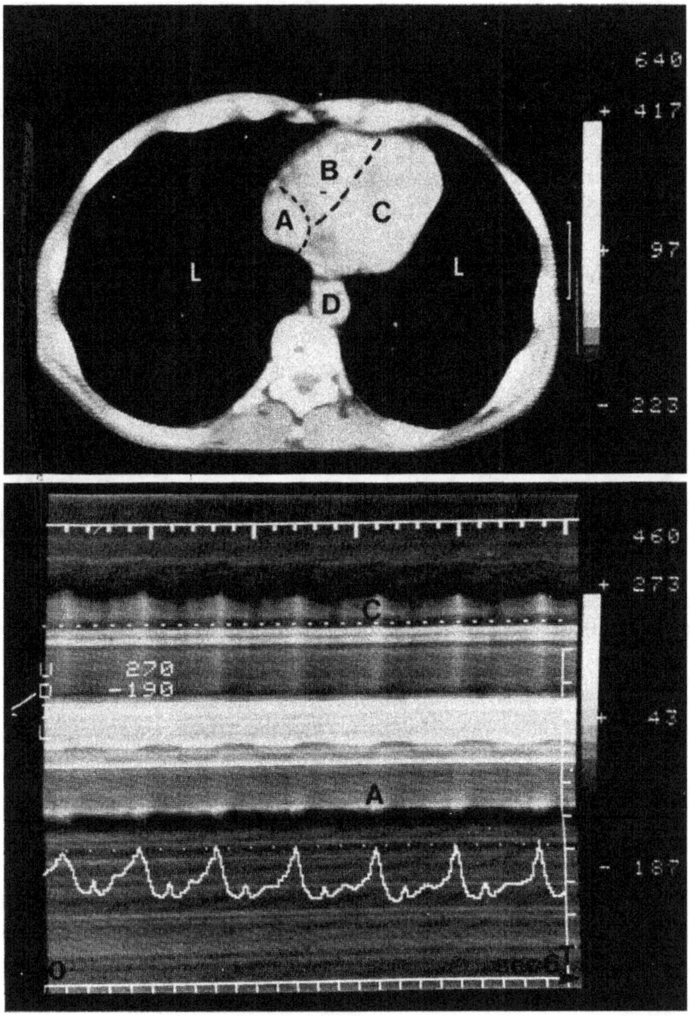

Fig. 32. a Reference CT scan related to Figs. 32b and 33. The "chronogram" was obtained in this sectional plane. *A*, right atrium; *B*, right ventricle; *C*, left ventricle; *D*, descending aorta, *L*, lung parenchyma. **b** Digital frequent absorption profile over 6 s (*T*). The pulsations of heart structures (Fig. 32a) are readily recognizable, also the density modulation of the left ventricle (*C*), which is shown by the histogram curve

means that 250 profiles can be recorded within 5 s; the interval between two lines in this case is 20 ms. If the pulse repetition rate is reduced to 20 Hz or 10 Hz, it is possible to record an image in about 12 or 24 s, respectively, with a time discrimination of 50 ms and 100 ms, respectively. In the equipment under study, radiographic exposure times of 5, 10, 12, 24 and 48 s can be preselected, thus making temporal differentiations of 20 ms to 200 ms per line possible – a spectrum which, in our experience, permits the adequate detection of major changes in density in various structures of the body.

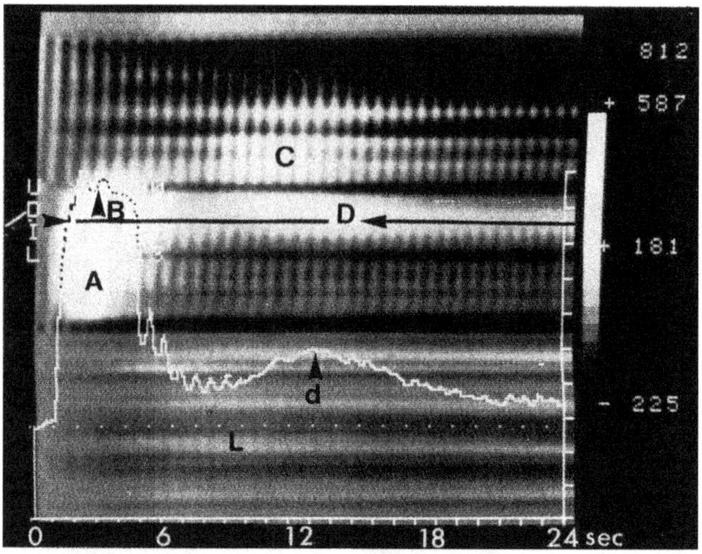

Fig. 33. Transmission profile view of the plane shown in Fig. 32a, following an intravenous bolus injection of 50 ml Rayvist 300 (Schering AG). The temporal discrimination of the passage of contrast material in the right atrium (*A*), the right ventricle (*B*) – with the peak of the histogram –, lung parenchyma (*L*), left ventricle (*C*) and descending aorta (*D*) with lower histogram peak (*d*) can readily be distinguished. Exposure time: 24 s (*abscissa*)

Applications of this recording technique are

1. Modulation of the transmission profile by the pulsation of the heart and blood vessels

If such a sequence of transmission profiles is recorded for the heart or pulsating blood vessels, the density modulations induced by the pulsation are readily recognizable. This high-frequency recording (Fig. 32) permits a high-resolution kinetic analysis (analysis of movement) which – in much more detail, but in only a narrow cross-section of the organ – corresponds to a kymographic picture.

If, on this view, a density histogram is superimposed, a sensitive measure for the motion amplitude and the shape of the detected organ contour over a number of actions is obtained. In a patient whose pulse rate is, for example, 60 per minute, at a radiographic exposure time of 5 s, five heart beats can be analysed, about 50 measuring profiles being recorded for each contraction.

A possible field of application might be the question as to the possible presence of dyskinesia of the heart (wall aneurysm, infarction, other pathology).

2. Modulation of the transmission profile by the respiratory and body movements

Each of these two-time-variable parameters may be considered merely as an interference factor.

3. Changes in the density profile due to the intravenous administration of contrast material

If a contrast medium bolus (for example, 50 ml of a 60% angiographic agent) is rapidly injected intravenously, it may be expected that during the transit of the contrast material in the sectional plane being imaged an increase in density will occur synchronously with the bolus form. In a preliminary study, we were able to confirm this assumption in the phantom (*Hübener* 1980, to be published). *Kruger* et al. (1981) also drew attention to such a possibility, and demonstrated the increase in density in animal experiments.

If the density profile is investigated in humans (Fig. 32), the radiographic view permits an analysis of the form and time of the contrast medium bolus in the region of the imaged vascular and organ structures. To facilitate orientation, it is always to be recommended that a computerized tomographic scan of the region of the body of interest to the examiner be obtained beforehand (Figs. 32, 33).

From these measurements, possibly in conjunction with subtraction views, information can be obtained about the distribution processes of the contrast material in the heart, blood vessels and organs, for example, in the presence of pathology or arteriovenous shunts, or, on the basis of a change in the form of a contrast medium bolus after its passage through the lungs or heart, conclusions may be drawn as to haemodynamic disturbances. Appropriate investigations into this question are presently being carried out.

3.5 Digital Radiography in Radiotherapeutic Treatment Planning in Patients with Malignant Tumours

In the radiotherapeutic treatment planning for tumour both of the body and of the head, the digital radiograph can be considered a valuable supplementation of the transversal sectional image obtained with the CT scanner; together, these two examinations can make the use of a therapy simulator superfluous. Where, previously, the third dimension was lacking for the CT establishment of the tumour or target volume, so that the coarse-rastered time-consuming production of secondary CT sections had to be employed, with the aid of digital radiography both planning and field checks together with field documentation can be optimized.

The standardized radiation treatments, which account for more than 80% of the therapeutic programme at the Medical Radiological Institute Tübingen (which treats more than 1600 patients annually) involve the following tumours in the body region:

1. Prostate gland and small pelvis
2. Urinary bladder, rectum and anus
3. Small pelvis in gynaecological, surgical patients
4. The parametria in cervical carcinoma with radium implants
5. Para-aortic region
6. Kidney beds in tumour nephrectomies
7. Oesophagus and cardia
8. The postoperative mamma
9. Bronchial/mediastinal tumours

The treatment modality, which, in the vast majority of cases is planned as moving-field therapy, is carried out exclusively on the basis of a combined com-

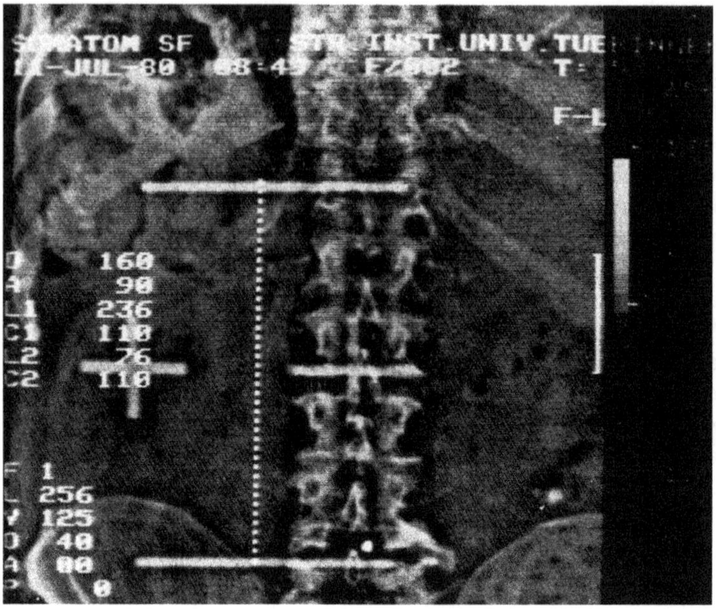

Fig. 34. Radiotherapeutic field identification in postoperative radiotherapy treatment of a left hypernephroid carcinoma (patient in the prone position). Marking of the middle of the field and the centre of the field setting for a small-angle rotational treatment of the kidney bed. Length of field (measurement) 160 mm

puterized tomographic/digital radiographic establishment of the target volumes and field boundaries.

On the basis of the knowledge of the extension of the tumour, established either at surgery or by means of CT, a digital radiograph of the relevant region of the body is first made, in order to establish the upper and lower boundaries of the treatment field and the middle of the field with reference to the axial skeleton. The coordinates of these "markers" are measured and determine the length and centre of the treatment field. For marking these points of reference, they are identified with the aid of thin sectional aluminium, imaging in two planes by preparing a further digital radiograph (Fig. 34) and documented for the purpose of field checking.

The markers thus established are then tattooed on the skin. For the execution of the treatment planning, CT transversal scans are then obtained on a level with the field markers, which then serve the Physical Department as a basis for the computer-aided isodose calculation of the treatment plan – after determining the target volume cross section (*Metzger* et al. 1980).

For the advantageous longitudinal pendulum mode of treatment of the tumours in the facial region (*Metzger* et al. 1980), the digital radiograph also serves as an important aid for treatment planning, and, here, too, can again replace the coarse-raster secondary CT views.

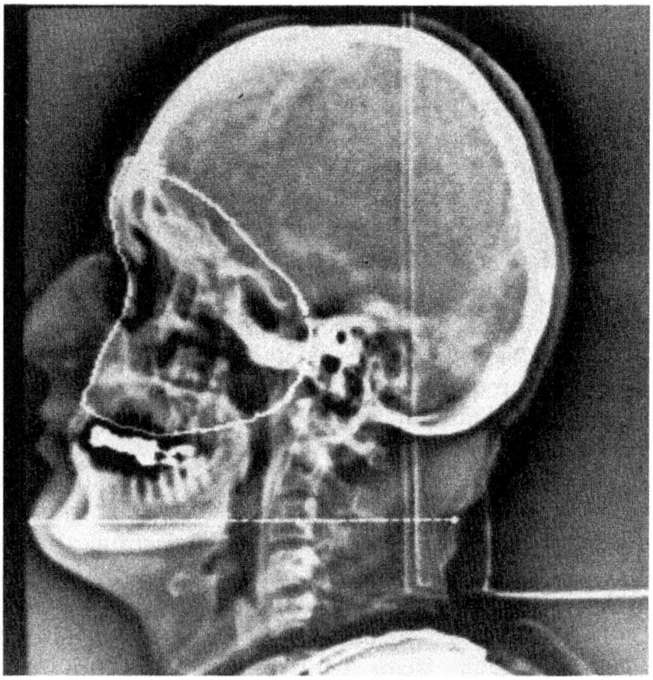

Fig. 35. Lateral radiograph of the head, with field marking for the radiotherapeutic treatment of an extensive carcinoma of the left maxillary sinus, with invasion of the orbit. Establishment of the field depth

In the case of tumours in the region of the orbits and facial sinuses, for which the longitudinal pendulum mode of treatment is indicated, following the localization of the tumour with prior computerized tomography, an anteroposterior and a lateral digital radiograph are obtained, in which, in addition to the possible bony destruction, the silhouette of the soft parts of the face are well delineated, the dimensions and "course" of which are, on account of the depth of the treatment field, important parameters for therapy planning. In the conventional film radiograph, this soft-tissue shadow is usually only inadequately visualized and also aberrant. With the marking of the target volume, the digital radiograph serves as a "measuring view" for the determination of the treatment modality and the extent of the field, as also for documentation (Fig. 35).

4 Summary

Computer-aided digital radiography as employed for radiodiagnostic purposes makes use of discrete countable (digital) picture elements in place of the quasi-continuous grey-scale spectrum of an X-ray film image. Although the coarsening of the image raster leads us to expect a reduction in the spatial resolution, with the aid of special measured data recording and the further digitized electronic processing of these data advantages may be expected for special diagnostic problems; these have been investigated in the present work.

Following a description of the data collection (measured value recording), the processing of the data and the representation of the image in digital radiography as can presently be carried out with the aid of a modified computerized tomographic scanner, the most important image-determining physical data are established.

In an investigation of the physical image-determining parameters, the radiation exposure in digital radiography is measured in the Alderson phantom [surface (skin) dose, emission dose, gonadal dose and scattered radiation] and comparisons are made with conventional film radiography.

The extremely low radiation dose (in the abdominal region less than 1% of the conventional film radiograph), the virtual absence of scattered radiation effects in the image, the total absence of distortion, the rapid examination of large areas of the body, the fact that incorrect exposures cannot be made, a spectrum of differentiable attenuation values that is ten times as large as that of the conventional radiograph and, finally, the possibility of electronically storing the radiographs are the decisive advantages of this imaging procedure. The possibilities of image reconstruction using various mathematical algorithms are examined and, by way of an example, the effects of electronic image manipulation described. An important image-determining factor is the relationship between the recognizable object size and object contrast, which, in a series of measurements, is determined as a contrast-detail diagram, and compared with the conventional radiographic film technique and the computerized tomographic scan. It is shown that digital radiography offers decisive advantages for objects that are larger than 1.5 mm in diameter and of low contrast (for example, faint circumscribed lesions in the lungs), while the conventional film radiograph proves clearly superior in the case of small objects with large contrast (for example, the spongy bone, the mucous membrane in the double contrast technique), although it must be admitted that, in the latter case, the radiation exposure to the patient is much higher.

An examination of the transmission linearity is followed by an investigation into the influence of object movements on the imaging quality which, at the relatively long exposure time of 10 s, is of considerable significance; it can be shown that all the physiological body (or organ) movements have only a small influence on the quality of the digital radiographic image, and that the image-producing X-ray pulse technique (2-ms duration) prevents any unsharpness of the radiograph. In the case of the heart, this type of data collecting leads to an image similar to that obtained with kymography.

Important possibilities of error and artefacts are discussed, and the invariable dose output as the decisive limiting factor in the examination of adipose patients is determined; in such patients, an inadequate signal-to-noise ratio can prevent the production of a satisfactory image quality.

The physical image transmission data are discussed and used as a basis for a consideration of the imaging properties of digital radiography to be expected in clinical application. Possible improvements for autonomic digital radiographic installations suggested by the results of the measurements, and also additional pointers for modifications to the data collecting and processing system, point up the possible perspectives of this technology.

Initial experience with this new technique is discussed in the clinical section, which is based on the evaluation of more than 1500 digital radiographs, mainly of the chest. In sample comparative images, the normal structures visualized in the digital radiograph and the conventional film radiograph are compared and the efficacy of the digital technique demonstrated on the basis of major pathology. It is seen that the exemplary radiographic images are capable of reproducing only a small portion of the overall information contained within the total data of a digital radiograph.

Besides the low radiation exposure to the patient and the large "range" of contrast in the radiograph in the chest area, the good representation of the mediastinal pleural reflections, the trachea together with the main bronchi and also the detectability of faint pulmonary shadows may be considered important advantages. In the abdominal area, the digital radiograph can provide all the important information of the "plain abdominal film", without the risk of producing an incorrectly exposed image, and at a minimum radiation burden. So far, the use of contrast materials in digital radiography is of very restricted value, since both in oral and in rectal contrast medium administration (mucous membranes) and in intravascular administration (vascular lesions), the digital diagnostic technique is, as yet, inadequate; the ease of production of subtraction views and the high density resolution, coupled with a reduction in the amount of contrast material needed, however, strongly suggest the usefulness of contrast medium applications for a future form of digital radiography.

An important indication for digital radiography is shown for the emergency diagnostic examination of polytraumatized patients. The rapid "sure-fire exposure" examination of large areas of the body can detect the pathological findings that are important with respect to emergency treatment [fractures with displacement of the fragments, pneumothorax] with a high degree of certainty, and without the usual delay. The experience reported in a study by *Curtis* (1979) is discussed.

A brief discussion is also presented of an innovative, high-frequency radiographic technique, carried out for the first time, and involving a *single* narrow section through the body, and the first such "chronograms" are presented with examples. With exposures of a selected transversal section of the body, repeatable using up to 50 X-ray pulses per second, it is probable that very rapid movements or changes in density (after the administration of contrast material) may be detected and subjected to a quantitative analysis.

Finally, the use of digital radiography in conjunction with computerized tomographic scanning in the field of radiotherapeutic treatment planning is described. At the present time, this combination of the two radiographic techniques has already become the standard of treatment planning at the Medical Radiological Institute at Tübingen, and will replace the formerly usual methods in the case of tumours of the trunk – in the main the use of therapy simulators.

Acknowledgements. I am particularly grateful to Dr. W. Kalender of Siemens A.G., Erlangen for technical advice and support.

References

Ayella RJ (1978) Radiologic management of the massively traumatized patient. Williams & Wilkins, Baltimore, pp 1–4

Baker HL Jr (1981) Screening for brain lesions with digital radiography of the head using a CT scanner. J Comp Assist Tomogr 5/1:54–59

Brody WR, Macovski A, Lehman L, DiBianca FA, Volz O, Edelheit LS (1980) Intravenous angiography using scanned projection radiography: Preliminary investigation of a new method. Invest Radiol 15/3:220–223

Curtis DJ, Ayella RJ, Whitley J, Moser RP, Rugh KS (1979) Digital Radiology in Trauma Using Small-Dose exposure. Radiology 132:587–591

Foley WD, Lawson TL, Scanlon GT, Heeschen RC, DiBianca F (1979) Digital radiography of the chest using a computed tomography instrument. Radiology 133:231–234

Hübener K-H (1980) Digitale Radiographie – Möglichkeiten und Perspektiven einer neuen radiologischen Technik. Habilitationsarbeit, Universität Tübingen 1980

Hübener K-H, Kalender W, Metzger HOFJ (to be published) Fast digital recording of X-ray attenuation profiles: A preliminary evaluation. Radiology

Hübener K-H, Klott K-J (1980) "Statisches" und dynamisches Kontrastmittelenhancement der Körperstamm-Computertomographie. Fortschr Röntgenstr 133/4:347–354

Katragadda CS, Fogel SR, Cohen G, Wagner LK, Morgan C, Handel SF, Amtey SR, Lester RG (1979) Digital radiography using a computed tomography instrument. Radiology 133:83–87

Kramann B, Christen N (1978) Die intravenöse Arteriographie im Xeroxbild: Eine nichtinvasive Methode zur Darstellung peripherer Gefäße. Fortschr. Röntgenstr. 128/3:319–323

Kruger RA, Anderson RE, Koehler PR, Nelson JA, Sorenson JA, Morgan T (1981) A Method for the noninvasive evaluation of cardiovascular dynamics using a digital radiographic device. Radiology 139:301–305

Lawson TL, Fooley WD, Imray TJ, Stewart ET, Wilson CR, Youker JE (1980) Abdominal computed radiography: Evaluation of low-contrast lesions. Invest Radiol 15/3:215–219

Metzger H, Hübener K-H, Klott K (1980) Bestrahlungsplanung mit computerisierter digitaler Radiographie. Strahlentherapie 156:684–688

Stein JA (1975) X-ray imaging with a scanning beam. Radiology 117:713–716

Stenberg I, Finby N, Evans JA (1959) A safe and practical intravenous method for abdominal aortography, peripheral arteriography and cerebral arteriography. Amer J Roentgenol 82:758–771

Stieve FE (ed) (1966) Bildgüte in der Radiologie. Gustav Fischer Verlag, Stuttgart

GPSR Compliance
The European Union's (EU) General Product Safety Regulation (GPSR) is a set of rules that requires consumer products to be safe and our obligations to ensure this.

If you have any concerns about our products, you can contact us on

ProductSafety@springernature.com

In case Publisher is established outside the EU, the EU authorized representative is:

Springer Nature Customer Service Center GmbH
Europaplatz 3
69115 Heidelberg, Germany

www.ingramcontent.com/pod-product-compliance
Lightning Source LLC
Chambersburg PA
CBHW061213240926
51846CB00006B/1217
* 9 7 8 3 6 4 2 9 5 3 9 2 7 *